Ventricular Arrhythmias in Apparently Normal Hearts

Editors

FRANK M. BOGUN
THOMAS C. CRAWFORD
RAKESH LATCHAMSETTY

CARDIAC ELECTROPHYSIOLOGY CLINICS

www.cardiacEP.theclinics.com

Consulting Editors
RANJAN K. THAKUR
ANDREA NATALE

September 2016 • Volume 8 • Number 3

ELSEVIER

1600 John F. Kennedy Boulevard • Suite 1800 • Philadelphia, Pennsylvania, 19103-2899

http://www.theclinics.com

CARDIAC ELECTROPHYSIOLOGY CLINICS Volume 8, Number 3
September 2016 ISSN 1877-9182, ISBN-13: 978-0-323-46252-5

Editor: Lauren Boyle
Developmental Editor: Susan Showalter

Cardiac Electrophysiology Clinics (ISSN 1877-9182) is published quarterly by Elsevier Inc., 360 Park Avenue South, New York, NY 10010-1710. Months of issue are March, June, September, and December. Subscription prices are $205.00 per year for US individuals, $318.00 per year for US institutions, $225.00 per year for Canadian individuals, $359.00 per year for Canadian institutions, $285.00 per year for international individuals, $384.00 per year for international institutions and $100.00 per year for US, Canadian and international students/residents. To receive student/resident rate, orders must be accompanied by name of affiliated institution, date of term, and the signature of program/residency coordinator on institution letterhead. Orders will be billed at individual rate until proof of status is received. Foreign air speed delivery is included in all Clinics subscription prices. All prices are subject to change without notice. **POSTMASTER:** Send address changes to Cardiac Electrophysiology Clinics, Elsevier Health Sciences Division, Subscription Customer Service, 3251 Riverport Lane, Maryland Heights, MO 63043. **Customer Service: 1-800-654-2452 (US and Canada). From outside of the US and Canada, call 314-477-8871. Fax: 314-447-8029. E-mail: JournalsCustomerService-usa@elsevier.com (for print support); JournalsOnlineSupport-usa@elsevier.com (for online support).**

Reprints. For copies of 100 or more of articles in this publication, please contact the Commercial Reprints Department, Elsevier Inc., 360 Park Avenue South, New York, NY 10010-1710. Tel.: 212-633-3874; Fax: 212-633-3820; E-mail: reprints@elsevier.com.

Cardiac Electrophysiology Clinics is covered in *MEDLINE/PubMed (Index Medicus)*.

Contributors

CONSULTING EDITORS

RANJAN K. THAKUR, MD, MPH, MBA, FACC, FHRS
Professor of Medicine and Director, Arrhythmia Service, Thoracic and Cardiovascular Institute, Sparrow Health System, Michigan State University, Lansing, Michigan

ANDREA NATALE, MD, FACC, FHRS
Texas Cardiac Arrhythmia Institute, St. David's Medical Center, Austin, Texas; Dell Medical School, University of Texas, Austin, Texas; MetroHealth Medical Center, Case Western Reserve University School of Medicine, Cleveland, Ohio; Division of Cardiology, Stanford University, Stanford, California; Electrophysiology and Arrhythmia Services, California Pacific Medical Center, San Francisco, California; Division of Cardiovascular Diseases, Scripps Clinic, La Jolla, California

EDITORS

FRANK M. BOGUN, MD
Associate Professor of Internal Medicine, Division of Cardiovascular Medicine, Cardiovascular Center, University of Michigan, Ann Arbor, Michigan

RAKESH LATCHAMSETTY, MD
Assistant Professor, Division of Cardiovascular Medicine, Cardiovascular Center, University of Michigan, Ann Arbor, Michigan

THOMAS C. CRAWFORD, MD, FACC, FHRS
Assistant Professor, Department of Internal Medicine, The University of Michigan Health System, Ann Arbor, Michigan

AUTHORS

SAMUEL J. ASIRVATHAM, MD
Division of Cardiovascular Diseases, Department of Medicine; Division of Pediatric Cardiology, Department of Pediatric and Adolescent Medicine, Mayo Clinic, Rochester, Minnesota

ARNAUD DENIS, MD
Department of Electrophysiology and Cardiac Pacing, Hôpital Cardiologique du Haut Lévêque, Pessac, France

DENISE AUBERSON, MD
Department of Medicine, Pennsylvania Hospital, University of Pennsylvania Health System, Philadelphia, Pennsylvania

NICOLAS DERVAL, MD
Department of Electrophysiology and Cardiac Pacing, Hôpital Cardiologique du Haut Lévêque, Pessac, France

KENNETH ELLENBOGEN, MD, FHRS
Kontos Professor of Medicine; Chairman,
Division of Cardiology, VCU Pauley Heart
Center, Medical College of Virginia, Virginia
Commonwealth University School of Medicine,
Richmond, Virginia

MICHEL HAISSAGUERRE, MD
Department of Electrophysiology and Cardiac
Pacing, Hôpital Cardiologique du Haut
Lévêque, Pessac, France

MELEZE HOCINI, MD
Department of Electrophysiology and Cardiac
Pacing, Hôpital Cardiologique du Haut
Lévêque, Pessac, France

NYNKE HOFMAN, PhD
Department of Clinical Genetics, Academic
Medical Center, Amsterdam, The Netherlands

PIERRE JAIS, MD
Department of Electrophysiology and Cardiac
Pacing, Hôpital Cardiologique du Haut
Lévêque, Pessac, France

JOSÉ JALIFE, MD
Professor of Internal Medicine and The Cyrus
and Jane Farrehi Professor of Cardiovascular
Research; Professor of Molecular & Integrative
Physiology; Director, Center for Arrhythmia
Research, North Campus Research Complex,
University of Michigan, Ann Arbor, Michigan

ROY M. JOHN, MBBS, MD, PhD
Assistant Professor, Department of Medicine,
Brigham and Women's Hospital, Harvard
Medical School, Boston, Massachusetts

SURAJ KAPA, MD
Division of Cardiovascular Diseases,
Department of Medicine, Mayo Clinic,
Rochester, Minnesota

GEORGE J. KLEIN, MD, FHRS
Professor, Division of Cardiology, Department
of Medicine, Western University, London,
Ontario, Canada

PETER LEONG-SIT, MD, MSc, FHRS
Associate Professor of Medicine, Division of
Cardiology, Department of Medicine, Western
University, London, Ontario, Canada

JEFFREY LUEBBERT, MD
Section of Cardiac Electrophysiology,
Cardiovascular Division, Department of
Medicine, Pennsylvania Hospital, University of
Pennsylvania Health System, Philadelphia,
Pennsylvania

FRANCIS MARCHLINSKI, MD
Richard T. and Angela Clark President's
Distinguished Professor; Director of Cardiac
Electrophysiology, University of Pennsylvania
Health System, Philadelphia, Pennsylvania

JOSEPH E. MARINE, MD, FACC, FHRS
Associate Professor of Medicine;
Vice-Director, Division of Cardiology, Johns
Hopkins University School of Medicine,
Baltimore, Maryland

YOAV MICHOWITZ, MD
Department of Cardiology, Tel Aviv Sourasky
Medical Center, Sackler School of Medicine,
Tel Aviv University, Tel Aviv, Israel

JOSHUA D. MOSS, MD
Center for Arrhythmia Care, Heart and Vascular
Center, The University of Chicago Medicine,
Chicago, Illinois

NIYADA NAKSUK, MD
Division of Cardiovascular Diseases,
Department of Medicine, Mayo Clinic,
Rochester, Minnesota

RAPHAEL ROSSO, MD
Department of Cardiology, Tel Aviv Sourasky
Medical Center, Sackler School of Medicine,
Tel Aviv University, Tel Aviv, Israel

FREDERIC SACHER, MD
Department of Electrophysiology and Cardiac
Pacing, Hôpital Cardiologique du Haut
Lévêque, Pessac, France

ALI KAZEMI SAEID, MD
Division of Cardiology, Department of
Medicine, Western University, London,
Ontario, Canada

MELVIN SCHEINMAN, MD
University of California San Francisco, San
Francisco, California

ASHOK J. SHAH, MD
Cardio Vascular Services, South Consulting Suites, Peel Health Campus, Mandurah, Western Australia, Australia

WILLIAM G. STEVENSON, MD
Professor, Department of Medicine, Brigham and Women's Hospital, Harvard Medical School, Boston, Massachusetts

RAPHAEL SUNG, MD
Community Hospital of the Monterey Peninsula, Monterey, California

ALEX Y. TAN, MD
Assistant Professor of Medicine, Electrophysiology Section, Division of Cardiology, Hunter Holmes McGuire VA Medical Center; VCU Pauley Heart Center, Medical College of Virginia, Virginia Commonwealth University School of Medicine, Richmond, Virginia

RODERICK TUNG, MD
Center for Arrhythmia Care, Heart and Vascular Center, The University of Chicago Medicine, Chicago, Illinois

SAMI VISKIN, MD
Department of Cardiology, Tel Aviv Sourasky Medical Center, Sackler School of Medicine, Tel Aviv University, Tel Aviv, Israel

ARTHUR A.M. WILDE, MD, PhD
Professor, Department of Cardiology, Academic Medical Center, Amsterdam, The Netherlands

tachycardia, short QT syndrome, and early repolarization syndrome. This article reviews the clinical electrophysiological management of PMVT/VF in a structurally normal heart affected with these disorders.

Exercise-induced Ventricular Tachycardia/Ventricular Fibrillation in the Normal Heart: Risk Stratification and Management

Yoav Michowitz, Sami Viskin, and Raphael Rosso

Exercise-induced ventricular tachycardia (VT) rarely occurs in the absence of organic heart disease. Idiopathic monomorphic VT has an excellent prognosis. The main aspect of the risk stratification process is recognizing subtle forms of organic heart disease, particularly arrhythmogenic right ventricular cardiomyopathy. Exercise-induced polymorphic VT is potentially malignant. Exercise-induced polymorphic VT has also been seen in mitral valve prolapse. Some patients with stable coronary disease, and even healthy athletes, sometimes have short bursts of polymorphic VT during exercise tests but these arrhythmias are usually not reproducible during repeated testing and have unknown long-term clinical significance.

Dynamics and Molecular Mechanisms of Ventricular Fibrillation in Structurally Normal Hearts

José Jalife

Ventricular fibrillation (VF) is the most severe cardiac rhythm disturbance and one of the most important immediate causes of sudden cardiac death. In the structurally normal heart, a small number of stable reentrant sources, perhaps 1 or 2, underlie the mechanism of VF, and the stabilization of the sources, their frequency, and the complexity of the turbulent waves they generate depend on the expression, spatial distribution, and intermolecular interactions of the 2 most important ion channels that control cardiac excitability: the inward rectifier potassium channel, Kir2.1, and the alpha subunit of the main cardiac sodium channel, $Na_V1.5$.

Ventricular Arrhythmias in Apparently Normal Hearts: Who Needs an Implantable Cardiac Defibrillator?

Alex Y. Tan and Kenneth Ellenbogen

Idiopathic ventricular tachycardia is often considered a benign form of ventricular arrhythmia in patients without apparent structural heart disease. However, a subset of patients may develop malignant ventricular arrhythmias and present with syncope and sudden cardiac arrest. Survivors of cardiac arrest are candidates for implantable cardiac defibrillators (ICDs). The indications for ICDs in patients with less than a full-blown cardiac arrest presentation but with electrocardiographically high-risk ectopy features remain uncertain. This article addresses some of the uncertainties and pitfalls in ICD risk stratification in this patient group and explores potential mechanisms for malignant conversion of benign premature ventricular complexes to sustained arrhythmia.

Sustained Ventricular Tachycardia in Apparently Normal Hearts: Ablation Should Be the First Step in Management

Joshua D. Moss and Roderick Tung

Patients without structural heart disease tend to have fewer morphologies of ventricular tachycardia, with automaticity and triggered activity a more common mechanism than re-entry associated with extremely low risk of sudden death. Ablation can be curative in patients with a single morphology of ventricular tachycardia that is focal in origin, particularly in patients without overt structural heart disease. There are limited data in secondary prevention implantable cardioverter defibrillator literature to support the routine implementation of implantable cardioverter defibrillator in normal hearts. Antiarrhythmic drugs have not been shown to reduce all-cause mortality in patients with and without structural heart disease.

Sustained monomorphic ventricular tachycardia or repetitive premature ventricular complexes can be seen in patients with structurally normal hearts. Among these types of patients, the prognosis is predominantly benign and the treatment mostly focused on elimination of symptoms rather than improving survival or reduction of mortality. This article focuses on the pharmacologic options for management and compares them with invasive options. Based on the current literature, we demonstrate that medical therapies should be used as first-line management and favored over invasive therapies. Understanding the arrhythmia mechanism is critical in choosing the appropriate medication among the wide variety of antiarrhythmic drugs available.

CARDIAC ELECTROPHYSIOLOGY CLINICS

THE CLINICS ARE AVAILABLE ONLINE!
Access your subscription at:
www.theclinics.com

Foreword
A Matter of Definition

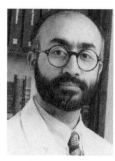 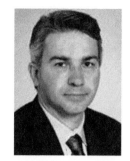

Ranjan K. Thakur, MD, MPH, MBA, FHRS   Andrea Natale, MD, FACC, FHRS

Consulting Editors

By definition, "normal" hearts shouldn't give rise to significant ventricular arrhythmias. By using the word "apparently" in the title of this issue, the editors have emphasized that hearts giving rise to ventricular arrhythmias may not be "normal," but appear normal. Some others may use the moniker, "structurally normal," or some other qualifier to convey the same concept when classifying these arrhythmias. In this context, "normal" implies that there is no obvious heart disease based on ventricular function, absence of structural abnormalities discernible on an echocardiogram, or evident ischemia by stress testing or coronary angiography. Some authors would exclude from this group patients with abnormal ECGs, such as long- or short-QT syndromes and Brugada syndrome, as well as patients with abnormalities seen on a cardiac MRI, such as right ventricular dysplasia or sarcoid heart disease.

"Normal" hearts may be seen in up to 10% of patients presenting with significant ventricular arrhythmias. Our understanding of these disorders has evolved considerably over the last three decades, and the arrhythmias that may be included in this discussion depend on how wide a net one wants to cast and how one wishes to categorize them. The editors have decided to focus on commonly encountered arrhythmias in clinical practice: outflow tract arrhythmias, papillary muscle arrhythmias, fascicular tachycardias, nonsustained-, polymorphic-, and exercise-induced arrhythmias, as well as the role of genetic testing, ICDs, and the role of medical therapy and catheter ablation.

We congratulate Drs Frank M. Bogun, Thomas C. Crawford, and Rakesh Latchamsetty for editing this issue of *Cardiac Electrophysiology Clinics* and for providing a practical discussion of "arrhythmias in apparently normal hearts," based on contemporary understanding and current clinical approaches. They have drawn from leaders in electrophysiology to discuss these important arrhythmias in order to provide authoritative reviews. We hope that the readers will find the issue helpful in broadening their understanding of these arrhythmias.

Ranjan K. Thakur, MD, MPH, MBA, FHRS
Sparrow Thoracic and Cardiovascular Institute
Michigan State University
1200 East Michigan Avenue, Suite 580
Lansing, MI 48912, USA

Andrea Natale, MD, FACC, FHRS
Texas Cardiac Arrhythmia Institute
Center for Atrial Fibrillation at
St. David's Medical Center
1015 East 32nd Street, Suite 516
Austin, TX 78705, USA

E-mail addresses:
thakur@msu.edu (R.K. Thakur)
andrea.natale@stdavids.com (A. Natale)

http://dx.doi.org/10.1016/j.ccep.2016.07.002
1877-9182/16/© 2016 Published by Elsevier Inc.

cardiacEP.theclinics.com

Preface

Ventricular Arrhythmias in Apparently Normal Hearts

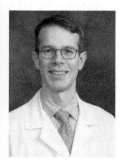 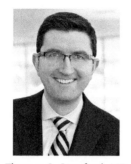 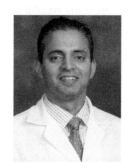

Frank M. Bogun, MD   Thomas C. Crawford, MD   Rakesh Latchamsetty, MD

Editors

The diagnosis of ventricular arrhythmia in patients with structurally normal hearts is often accompanied by a sense of trepidation among patients as well as treating physicians. Unlike patients with a history of myocardial infarction or nonischemic cardiomyopathy, where the treatment strategy tends to be more obvious, patients with structurally normal hearts and ventricular arrhythmias tend to be underrepresented in large clinical trials. Many have a benign prognosis, but this is not uniformly true. Epidemiologic studies have shown frequent premature ventricular complexes (PVCs) to be associated with a worse prognosis. Malignant variants of PVCs may induce ventricular fibrillation even in an apparently normal heart, a term often used to indicate preserved left ventricular function. Rigorous exclusion of structural heart disease has not been performed in many of these studies.

In order to exclude the presence of structural heart disease, the clinical evaluation of patients with PVCs and ventricular tachycardia (VT) should consist of a complete history, physical exam, 12-lead electrocardiogram, and 12-lead Holter monitor to define the morphology and frequency of the PVCs. Occasionally, an event monitor is helpful in symptomatic patients. An echocardiogram, exercise stress test, and, where appropriate, advanced imaging with cardiac magnetic resonance, cardiac computerized tomography, and PET are revealing of more subtle abnormalities. Some patients may require an invasive electrophysiologic study to assess for inducible VT, while in others, genetic testing is more appropriate. Whether the heart is considered "normal" depends in part on how sensitive the employed diagnostic tools are. Sometimes ventricular arrhythmias in the form of PVCs or nonsustained VT are the only manifestation of a more ominous condition, a type of "forme fruste."

In this set of articles written by some of the greatest experts in the field, we seek to approach patients with apparently normal hearts from the

Card Electrophysiol Clin 8 (2016) xv–xvi
http://dx.doi.org/10.1016/j.ccep.2016.07.001
1877-9182/16/© 2016 Published by Elsevier Inc.

perspective of the clinician charged with deciding how to best manage these patients. Risk stratification is an essential aspect of this task. Our contributors discuss diagnostic studies and best approaches, utilizing medical management, ablation, and device therapy.

We hope that you will find this issue helpful in your day-to-day evaluation of patients with ventricular arrhythmias and a structurally normal heart.

Frank M. Bogun, MD
Division of Cardiovascular Medicine
Cardiovascular Center
University of Michigan
1500 East Medical Center Drive
SPC 5853
Ann Arbor, MI 48109-5853, USA

Thomas C. Crawford, MD
Division of Cardiovascular Medicine
Cardiovascular Center
University of Michigan
1500 East Medical Center Drive
SPC 5853
Ann Arbor, MI 48109-5853, USA

Rakesh Latchamsetty, MD
Division of Cardiovascular Medicine
Cardiovascular Center
University of Michigan
1500 E Medical Center Drive
SPC 5856
Ann Arbor, MI 48109, USA

E-mail addresses:
fbogun@med.umich.edu (F.M. Bogun)
thomcraw@umich.edu (T.C. Crawford)
rakeshl@med.umich.edu (R. Latchamsetty)

Premature Ventricular Complexes in Apparently Normal Hearts

Jeffrey Luebbert, MD[a], Denise Auberson, MD[a],
Francis Marchlinski, MD[b],*

KEYWORDS

- PVC-induced cardiomyopathy • Catheter ablation • Idiopathic ventricular fibrillation

KEY POINTS

- Although generally considered benign, epidemiologic studies have consistently shown PVCs to be associated with a worse prognosis and higher morbidity and mortality than those patients without PVCs.
- Diagnostic evaluation in the patient with PVCs and no known structural heart disease should consist of complete history; physical; 12-lead ECG; 24-hour Holter monitor; echocardiogram; and where appropriate advanced imaging with exercise stress test, cardiac MRI, cardiac PET scan, and endocardial voltage mapping to exclude structural heart disease, define the morphology and frequency of the PVCs, and if appropriate plan for ablation.
- Options for management for patients with PVCs include watchful waiting if asymptomatic and normal ejection fraction with at least yearly evaluation and echocardiography, β-blockers, calcium channel blockers, antiarrhythmic medications, or catheter ablation.
- Catheter ablation is potentially curative in patients with high-risk or malignant PVCs including PVC-induced ventricular fibrillation.
- Catheter ablation is superior to medical therapy for PVC-induced cardiomyopathy and after successful ablation most show improvement in EF after 3 to 12 months.

PREMATURE VENTRICULAR COMPLEXES IN STRUCTURALLY NORMAL HEARTS: PRESENTATION AND DETECTION

Premature ventricular complexes (PVCs), also referred to as ventricular premature beats or ventricular extrasystoles, are common and prevalent in individuals with and without structural heart disease. The prevalence of PVCs depends on the characteristics and comorbidities of the population, the method by which the population is studied, and the duration of observation. In a review of healthy Air Force recruits with no known structural heart disease the prevalence of PVCs on surface electrocardiogram (ECG) was 2.4%.[1] When monitored for 24 hours with ambulatory Holter, the prevalence of PVCs reported in individuals without structural heart disease ranges from 40% to 100%.[2–6] Population studies, such as the Atherosclerosis Risk in Communities (ARIC) and a subset of the Multiple Risk Factor Intervention Trial (MRFIT), demonstrated a higher prevalence of PVCs in men than women, African Americans compared with white persons, and an increased

Disclosures: None.
[a] Department of Medicine, Pennsylvania Hospital, University of Pennsylvania Health System, 230 West Washington Square, Philadelphia, PA 19106, USA; [b] Perelman Center for Advanced Medicine, East Pavilion, 2nd Floor, 3400 Civic Center Boulevard, Philadelphia, PA 19104, USA
* Corresponding author.
E-mail address: Francis.Marchlinski@uphs.upenn.edu

Card Electrophysiol Clin 8 (2016) 503–514
http://dx.doi.org/10.1016/j.ccep.2016.04.001
1877-9182/16/$ – see front matter © 2016 Elsevier Inc. All rights reserved.

prevalence in individuals with hypertension. Increasing age was noted to be associated with higher PVC burden with a 34% increase for each 5-year increment increase in age.[5,7] The mechanism of PVCs in patients with a structurally normal heart seems to be cyclic adenosine monophosphate–mediated triggered activity.[8–10]

Symptoms

Symptoms are mild or absent in many patients; however, in some individuals symptoms are disabling. Common symptoms include palpitations and dizziness; frequently these symptoms may be caused by the PVC or the subsequent compensatory pause. The pause allows time for greater calcium uptake by the myocardium and a sinus beat following PVC is hypercontractile. Symptoms may be attributed to the PVC, the compensatory pause, hypercontractile sinus beat, or a combination of all. Other symptoms include lightheadedness and near syncope with the onset of ventricular bigeminy and a sudden decrement to one half of the hemodynamically effective heart rate (**Fig. 1**). A sensation that the heart has "stopped" or pulsation in the head or neck can be noted. Pulsation of the head or neck may correlate with the physical examination finding of "cannon" A waves because a PVC may trigger simultaneous contraction of the atria and ventricles and contraction of the atria against closed mitral and tricuspid valves. Symptoms of heart failure or abrupt syncope are concerning for high-risk forms of PVCs, such as those producing cardiomyopathy or PVC-induced ventricular fibrillation (VF) and should prompt further diagnostic evaluation.

Diagnostic Evaluation

Personal and family history should focus on excluding known structural heart disease including early coronary artery disease; previous myocardial infarction; valvular heart disease; and excluding any family history of inheritable conditions including channelopathies, hypertrophic cardiomyopathy, or arrhythmogenic right ventricular cardiomyopathy. Endocrine disorders, such as thyroid, adrenal, or pituitary abnormalities, may uncommonly precipitate or affect the burden of PVCs. A history of sarcoidosis in any organ system or obstructive sleep apnea may require further evaluation for structural heart disease. Social history should screen for illicit drug use and over-the-counter medications that may contain stimulant or sympathomimetic compounds. A full history of herbal medications with package inserts should be reviewed. Some patients may identify triggers in food or drink that correlate with increased burden of PVCs.

Diagnostic evaluation of patients with symptoms of PVCs should be directed at confirmation of PVC as a cause of symptoms, quantifying the daily burden as number or percent of all beats and determining the different morphologies of the PVCs. Initial evaluation should consist of a 12-lead ECG and ambulatory monitor of at least 24 hours, with longer duration if absence of symptoms during monitoring period. Patients with intermittent symptoms may need 30-day monitoring or rarely implantable loop recorder to document the presence of PVCs and correlation with symptoms. Patients should have transthoracic echocardiogram to identify significant structural heart disease. Additional imaging with cardiac MRI or cardiac PET scan may be considered in patients with multiple morphologies of PVCs or abnormal surface ECG to help identify such conditions as arrhythmogenic right ventricular dysplasia, amyloidosis, or cardiac sarcoidosis.[11,12] Treadmill stress testing allows characterization of morphology of PVCs, response

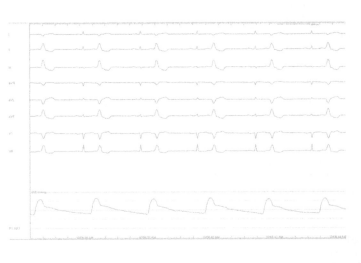

Fig. 1. Nonperfused PVC producing a sudden decrease in heart rate and presyncope. Surface ECG leads and arterial pressure tracing are shown.

of ectopy to catecholamines, and determination if the patient has provoked sustained or nonsustained ventricular tachycardia. Patients with nocturnal predominant burden of PVCs should be considered for evaluation of sleep apnea. Electrophysiology study is not generally necessary as part of the initial evaluation; however, it may be helpful in establishing diagnoses, such as arrhythmogenic right ventricular dysplasia or other infiltrative cardiomyopathy particularly, if used with bipolar and unipolar voltage mapping and cardiac biopsy.[13–16]

HIGH-RISK FEATURES/MALIGNANT

Although PVCs are common and are frequently believed to be benign, there are multiple studies showing higher risk for all-cause and cardiovascular mortality in patients without structural heart disease and PVCs. Population studies, such as the Framingham Heart study, MRFIT, and ARIC, have demonstrated PVCs to be an independent risk for death from coronary artery disease and sudden death, and are also associated with higher risk of all-cause mortality.[5,17,18]

Multiple factors may contribute to a worse prognosis in patients with PVCs. Frequent PVCs (defined as >1 PVC on a 10-second ECG or >30 in an hour) have been associated with increased risk for sudden cardiac death.[19] Investigators of the Cardiovascular Health Study prospectively examined the effect of PVC frequency on the risk of incident heart failure and mortality in 1139 subjects with a median follow up of 13 years. Subjects in the highest quartile of PVCS (0.123% to 17.7%) had a three-fold increase in the adjusted risk of left ventricular (LV) ejection fraction (EF) decline and a 48% and 31% relative risk increase of heart failure and death, respectively, when compared with subjects in the lowest quartile of PVCs (0.0% to

0.002%) (**Fig. 2**).[20] PVC polymorphisms may also portend worse outcomes. A cohort of 3351 Taiwanese adults with structurally normal hearts was followed for 10 years. Compared with monomorphic ectopy, those patients with multiple morphologies of PVCs had higher rates of mortality, all-cause hospitalization, risk for transient ischemic attack, new-onset atrial fibrillation, and new-onset heart failure.[21] Stroke risk is also increased in patients with PVCs. The ARIC study observed an incidence of ischemic stroke of 6.6% in patients with PVCs versus a 4.1% incidence of stoke in patients without PVCs (hazard ratio, 1.7; 95% confidence interval, 1.3–2.2).[5] The Reasons for Geographic and Racial Differences in Stroke (REGARDS) study followed 24,460 participants and noted presence of PVCs on baseline ECG was associated with a 38% relative risk of stroke as compared with patients without PVCs (hazard ratio, 1.4; 95% confidence interval, 1.1–1.8).[22] Whether PVCs are a direct cause of ischemic stroke or an associated marker of a higher risk for stroke has not yet been determined.

PREMATURE VENTRICULAR COMPLEX–INDUCED VENTRICULAR FIBRILLATION

There has been an increasing recognition of PVCs as a cause or trigger for VF.[23–26] In patients without structural heart disease PVCs causing VF have been documented from the His-Purkinje system, right ventricular outflow tract (RVOT), right ventricular anterior wall, LV papillary muscles, or left ventricular outflow tract (LVOT).[23–30] Recently VPCs from the moderator band were recognized as an additional trigger and a location that may be associated with late recurrence.[31] Idiopathic or PVC-induced VF in the absence of acute ischemia is rare with an estimated incidence of 5% of all cases of resuscitated sudden death but 23% of cases in

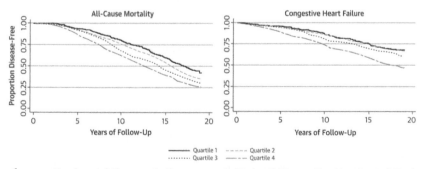

Fig. 2. Rates of congestive heart failure and all-cause mortality by PVC quartile. Unadjusted Kaplan-Meier estimates depicting incident congestive heart failure and mortality, as stratified by the percent of PVC count quartiles. Quartiles 1 through 4 represent PVC burdens of 0% to 0.002%, 0.002% to 0.011%, 0.011% to 0.123%, and 0.123% to 17.7%, respectively. (*From* Dukes JW, Dewland TA, Vittinghoff E, et al. Ventricular ectopy as a predictor of heart failure and death. J Am Coll Cardiol 2015;66(2):106; with permission.)

patients with preserved EF.[32,33] The mechanism of how PVCs induce VF in an otherwise structurally normal heart remains unclear. Early afterdepolarizations caused by inward calcium currents occur more readily in Purkinje cells.[34,35] Early afterdepolarizations may be potentiated via mechanical stretch, which leads to membrane depolarization and prolongation of the action potential.[36,37] The reason why distinct regions of the myocardium (papillary muscles, anterior right ventricular free wall, moderator band) seem to be common foci of these malignant varieties of PVCs may be related to greater activation of stretch-activated currents in these areas. However, proof of this concept in humans remains to be seen. Other possible mechanisms include a failure of a gating mechanism within the Purkinje network allowing for localized re-entry and autonomic interactions altering the dispersion of refractoriness to create the substrate necessary for idiopathic VF to occur.[31,38,39]

PREMATURE VENTRICULAR COMPLEX– INDUCED CARDIOMYOPATHY
Causes and Mechanism

PVCs may also be a direct cause of a reversible cardiomyopathy. The mechanism of this effect remains uncertain. There remains a dearth of animal models or prospective clinical data to elucidate a clear mechanism; therefore, the cause remains speculative. Possible mechanisms include alteration of membrane ionic currents and intracellular calcium handling, alteration in autonomic tone, and hemodynamics.[40–42] Ventricular dyssynchrony has been shown to compromise global mechanical cardiac function and lead to regional wall motion abnormalities with hypertrophy and alteration in blood flow.[43] PVCs may induce cardiomyopathy by impairment in radial, longitudinal, and circumferential strain, changes that seem to resolve completely with catheter ablation. These changes are not able to be detected by standard imaging and newer techniques, such as speckle tracking, may be needed to detect early presence of PVC cardiomyopathy.[44]

Risk Factors and Prevalence

Higher percentages of daily PVCs have been associated with PVC-induced cardiomyopathy; however, an absolute threshold has not been established. Authors have reported thresholds of 16%,[45] 24%,[46] or 26%[47] are more likely to contribute to cardiomyopathy; however, PVC-induced cardiomyopathy has been reported at lower daily burdens but rarely when less than 10%.[45,48,49] Given that the prevalence of

PVC-induced cardiomyopathy varies widely between studies with 6% to 7% of patients with greater than 10 PVCs per hour followed prospectively[45,48] to 38% of patients referred for catheter ablation,[49,50] PVC burden alone remains an imperfect tool for the prediction of those patients at risk for this condition. Recent studies have attempted to determine other risk markers for this condition that may allow identification of those patients at increased risk before the development of cardiomyopathy. Patients who are asymptomatic have been shown to have a higher risk for PVC-induced cardiomyopathy.[51,52] The duration of exposure to frequent PVCs is also associated with risk of PVC-induced cardiomyopathy and patients with long history of frequent PVCs have a higher risk.[53,54] Therefore, it is not surprising that those patients who are asymptomatic are at higher risk; their PVCs may be detected fortuitously after years of exposure to frequent PVC burden. Epicardial location has also been shown to be an independent risk factor for PVC-induced cardiomyopathy.[51,55] The wide QRS duration seen in epicardial PVCs may induce more dyssynchrony than those PVCs that conduct at least partially via the Purkinje network. Wide QRS duration without epicardial origin and non–outflow tract location of PVC have also been noted as risk factors for development of PVC-induced cardiomyopathy, with a QRS duration of at least 147 associated with increased risk.[49,53,55] Wide QRS duration during sinus rhythm has been recently reported to be a subtle manifestation of risk of progression to PVC-induced cardiomyopathy[49]; this concept of detection of markers to potentially intervene before development of cardiomyopathy deserves further study.

Treatment and Reversibility of Premature Ventricular Complex–Induced Cardiomyopathy

After successful ablation (with definition of acute success of an 80% reduction in the initial PVC burden) most patients demonstrate recovery in EF within 4 months.[56] In the same study 32% of patients demonstrated a prolonged resolution of cardiomyopathy with an average of 12 months and full recovery was delayed up to 45 months in one patient. In a comparison of patients undergoing PVC ablation with a control observation group continuing medical therapy, the likelihood of recovery of EF was 82% in the group undergoing ablation with no patients experiencing significant improvement in EF in the medical group at an average of 19 months of follow-up.[50] Only epicardial origin predicted delayed improvement in this study. Many but not all patients improve EF after ablation. Predictors of lack of improvement after successful ablation include PVC duration: PVCs with a more narrow duration (average, 153 milliseconds) were more likely to demonstrate reversibility of cardiomyopathy when compared with PVCs of longer duration (average, 179 milliseconds).[57] The wide QRS duration may be a marker that reflects the underlying severity of the cardiomyopathy and therefore may predict a lack of response to ablation. Complete elimination of all PVCs may not be necessary to demonstrate improvement. Both complete elimination and significant reduction to less than 80% of the preablation burden or typically less than 5000 PVCs a day may still lead to an improvement in EF after ablation.[58]

TREATMENT OPTIONS FOR PREMATURE VENTRICULAR COMPLEX

Patients with symptomatic PVCs or untoward effects of PVCs, such as PVC-induced cardiomyopathy and PVC-induced VF, should be offered treatment. In PVC-induced cardiomyopathy or PVC-induced VF, strong consideration should be given for early catheter ablation to reduce the burden of implantable cardioverter-defibrillator (ICD) shocks and potentially offer a long-term cure for PVC-induced cardiomyopathy. Consideration of treatment strategies depends on frequency and severity of symptoms, comorbidities, presence of monomorphic or pleomorphic varieties of PVCs, and patient preference. The optimal strategy for asymptomatic patients with significant PVCs without structural heart disease remains unknown. We recommend a comprehensive discussion with the patient about risks of progression to heart failure and consideration of all the treatment options with education on the side effects and possible complications of available therapies. A plan of close follow-up with monitoring for the development of LV structural changes (dilatation of decrease in diastolic function), decrease in systolic function, and symptoms of heart failure is appropriate. A yearly echocardiogram may be reasonable in most patients.

Medical Therapies

β-Blockade and calcium channel blockade

If an initial strategy of medication is pursued the first-line medication should be consideration of a β-blocker.[59] This medication is preferred as a first-line strategy given its safety and is generally well tolerated; however, it is modestly effective at suppressing PVCs.[60,61] The effectiveness of β-blockers to reduce symptoms and PVC burden is caused by the effect on β_1-adrenergic receptors to reduce intracellular cyclic adenosine monophosphate and thus reduce automaticity. A randomized, double blind, placebo-controlled trial of atenolol versus placebo in patients with structurally normal hearts demonstrated a decrease of PVCs from 24,000/24 hours to approximately 16,000/24 hours. However, neither the numeric decrease nor improvement in symptoms was statistically significant when compared with placebo.[60] If patients are intolerant to side effects of β-blockade (fatigue, marked sinus bradycardia, frequent bronchospastic exacerbation, erectile dysfunction) a calcium channel blocker may be considered. Nondihydropyidine calcium channel blockers (verapamil or diltiazem) may be effective in reducing burden of PVCs in patients intolerant of β-blockers with possible side effects of constipation, fatigue, bradycardia, and hypotension.

Antiarrhythmic medications

For patients with persistent symptoms despite calcium channel or β-blockade antiarrhythmic therapies may be considered. In patients without structural heart disease a 1C agent (flecainide or propafenone) is well tolerated and may be initiated safely in an outpatient setting. In patients without structural heart disease and greater than 100 PVCs an hour the burden of PVCs was reduced by greater than 70% in 91% of patients taking flecainide and 55% of patients taking mexilitine.[62] We usually start with a low dose and titrate to effect. Caution should be used with 1A and 1C agents in patients with structural heart disease with the possibility of increased risk of proarrhythmia and sudden death.[63] The use of the IC agents in setting of a suspected PVC-induced cardiomyopathy may be considered if significant structural abnormalities have been ruled out with cardiac MRI and/or detailed voltage mapping. Sotalol has been shown to reduce the PVC burden with a range of 8% to 67% including individuals with structural heart disease.[64–66] Serious side effects may occur with QT prolongation of significant concern and dose adjustments may be necessary in individuals of advanced age or impaired renal function. Amiodarone is effective at reducing the frequency of PVCs in patients with congestive heart failure when compared with placebo with additional benefit of improvement in EF with PVC suppression in some patients.[67] These results must be tempered with the need for long-term vigilance with follow-up and monitoring for toxicity of this medication.

Catheter Ablation

Indications

The most recent guidelines for catheter ablation for ventricular arrhythmias are from 2006. Catheter ablation for frequent symptomatic PVCs that have failed therapy with antiarrhythmic agents or in the setting where antiarrhythmics are not desired is given a IIa indication. Catheter ablation of PVCs, if the cause or a significant contributor of cardiomyopathy, currently carries IIb indication regardless of symptoms. An additional IIb indication is listed for those patients with malignant arrhythmias precipitated by single PVCs.[59] Since the publication of these guidelines, there has been a significant increase in the experience of the electrophysiologist in ablation of PVCs, improvement in technology, and dramatic increase in the published literature supporting PVC ablation in these clinical settings. Consideration of catheter ablation as a potential first-line therapy should be considered in patients with a presumed PVC cardiomyopathy to potentially halt progression or even reverse the abnormality. In addition, patients with PVC-induced VF should be considered for potentially first-line therapy with catheter ablation for the prevention of frequent therapies from an ICD.

Techniques for ablation

Principal techniques for catheter ablation start with localization with 12-lead ECG, activation mapping to localize the earliest source, and pacemapping. Algorithms have been used to help localize the source of the PVC to the RVOT or LVOT as a starting point for mapping and ablation. A right bundle branch block or left bundle branch block with transition in V2 morphology identifies an LV origin, and R wave progression that is later than V3 with a left bundle branch block QRS morphology points to an RVOT origin. For an left bundle branch block PVC morphology with a transition in V3, Betensky and colleagues[68] used a comparison with the sinus rhythm QRS transition and assessed the R wave amplitude in V2 as compared with that in sinus rhythm to localize the arrhythmia to the LVOT or RVOT. Mathematically this is expressed as $(R/R + S)_{VT}/(R/R + S)_{SR}$. A transition ratio of greater than 0.6 has a 95% sensitivity and 100% specificity to LVOT origin. For patients with frequent spontaneous ectopy we begin by mapping the RVOT unless localization by 12-lead ECG clearly suggests alternative location (right bundle branch block morphology at V1 suggesting LV origin or superiorly directed with late transition suggesting right ventricle or moderator band). We use multielectrode mapping

catheters with long or deflectable sheaths for stability to guide the ablation catheter (medium to large curl Agilis NxT or Lamp 90, St Jude Medical, St. Paul, MN), and continuous ECG recording. Use of phased-array intracardiac ultrasound with integrated three-dimensional mapping (Cartosound, Biosense Webster, Diamond Bar, CA) can assist in real-time integration of anatomy, catheter localization, and stability. For patients without significant ectopy β-adrenergic agonists (isoproterenol) may be used to attempt to provoke the arrhythmia. Occasionally atrial pacing can be used to provoke infrequent PVCs.

For those patients without significant ectopy despite β-agonist challenge pacemapping may be used to localize the site of ectopy with resolution estimated within 1.8 cm^2; however, the spatial resolution of this approach is inferior to activation mapping unless attention is given to the details of the QRS morphology. Similar pacemap QRS morphologies may be recorded up to 2 cm from the site of origin in 20% of patients.[69,70] By paying attention to all the subtleties of the QRS complex and using template matching algorithms that require greater than 90% to 95% match the specificity and localizing capability of pacemapping can be improved. PVCs originating from the RVOT generally have a local presystolic activation of greater than 20 milliseconds and these early sites produce a near perfect pacemap match. In the LVOT–aortic cusp region, pacemaps at sites of very early activation may not mimic VT; presumably the size of the virtual electrode with the higher output pacing required for capture may result in local capture with different QRS morphology. Occasionally by decreasing output to threshold values capture of the isolated muscle bundles responsible for the PVCs can result in identical pacemap-PVC QRS morphologies.

We frequently use irrigated tip catheters to overcome elevated temperatures at the tip of nonirrigated catheters limiting power delivery, particularly when ablating in the aortic root or coronary veins. We typically start with 20 W power and titrate to 40 W for 60 to 120 seconds. Suppression followed by early recurrence in an area should suggest a site of origin remote from the site of ablation and would prompt the operator to explore adjacent structures and reassess for earlier presystolic activity.

Complications of ablation

Complication rates have been reported to occur at approximately 5% for all complications, with major complications representing 2.4% to 3.0%.[71,72] Vascular access complications account for more than half of all complications. Valve disruption can rarely occur with ablation in the aortic cusp region. Cardiac perforation and tamponade have been reported at less than 1%. No deaths were reported in these series.[71,72]

Difficulties and limitations of ablation

Failure to eliminate PVCs acutely may occur from a variety of reasons. If unable to induce PVCs pacemapping may be pursued with success; however, if there are few PVCs it may be difficult to adjudicate a successful end point. It may be difficult to achieve catheter stability, particularly in mapping for PVC-induced VF, which may arise in small and highly mobile structures, such as the papillary muscles and moderator band.[26,31] Use of intracardiac echo may assist in monitoring for catheter stability; in addition the use of cryoablation may provide additional stability and allow for successful ablation when radiofrequency lesions fail (**Fig. 3**). PVC-induced cardiomyopathy may arise from difficult areas, such as the left ventricular summit, an area that is difficult to ablate because of overlying proximal branches of the coronary arteries and thick epicardial fat, and it may be difficult to obtain access to the origin of the PVC (**Fig. 4**). Possible solutions include mapping and ablation in the anterior intraventricular vein/great cardiac vein, lesions

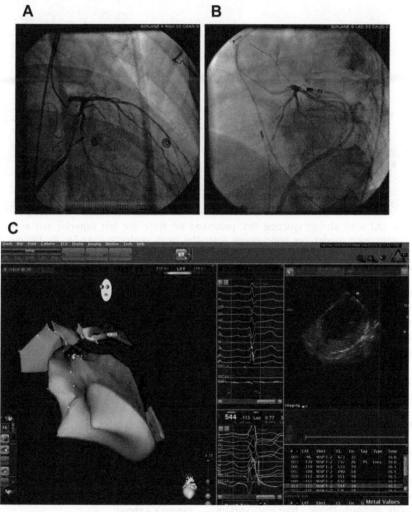

Fig. 3. Catheter position in initially unsuccessful PVC ablation in 50 year old with PVC-induced cardiomyopathy with EF 25%. Earliest site of activation was from the "left ventricular summit" with −30 ms pre-QRS with good unipolar electrogram; however, <2 mm away from bifurcation of left anterior descending and circumflex arteries (fluoroscopy 3A and 3B). (C) Electroanatomic image with intracardiac echo. Successful ablation was achieved from endocardial access directly across from earliest site with −20 ms pre-QRS activation with 35-W ablation lesions via irrigated ablation catheter with lesions of 60–300 seconds. After 3 months EF had normalized with no recurrence of PVCs.

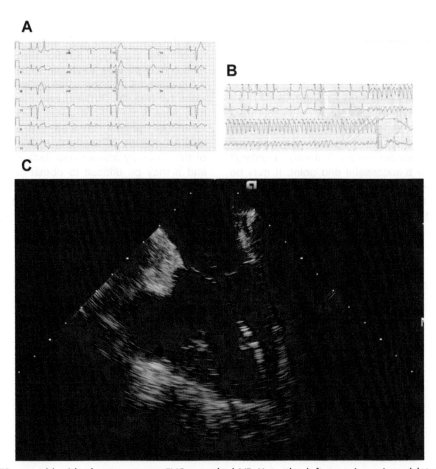

Fig. 4. A 52 year old with abrupt syncope PVC provoked VF. Note the left superior axis and late precordial transition consistent with moderator band origin near the right ventricle apex (*A, B*). Patient had recurrent episodes of PVC-induced VF; ablation was successful aided by deflectable sheaths and intracardiac echo documenting catheter location and lesion formation (*C*).

for extended duration and high wattage via the endocardium or adjacent aortic cusp region. True epicardial access with coronary angiography to guide for safety is rarely required. ECG clues suggesting a more apical and lateral segment of the summit away from the proximal coronaries can identify patients who may benefit from epicardial access.

Prognosis of right ventricular outflow tract ablation

When compared with medical therapy, a recent randomized trial showed the superiority of catheter ablation for treatment of RVOT PVCs. At 1 year of follow-up the recurrence rate of PVCs was 89% with antiarrhythmic therapy versus 21% for catheter ablation.[73]

Prognosis of premature ventricular complex–induced cardiomyopathy ablation

Success rates defined as greater than 80% reduction of PVC burden at 1 year post PVC ablation have varied with a range of 60% to 85%.[56,58,74] Of those patients with successful reduction in PVCs this portends likelihood of recovery of EF in a range of 47% to 100%.[56,74,75] A recent publication tested the safety of delaying ICD indicated for primary prevention of sudden death in medically maximized patients with frequent PVCs undergoing ablation. After successful ablation when followed out to 1 year 64% recovered EF to the extent that they would no longer qualify for ICD for primary prevention.[76] There were no sudden deaths or malignant arrhythmias observed in this group.

PROGNOSIS OF PREMATURE VENTRICULAR COMPLEX–INDUCED VENTRICULAR FIBRILLATION

A meta-analysis of 639 patients with idiopathic VF found a recurrence rate of VF of 31% with a mortality of 3.1% when followed for an average of 5.3 years.[77] The lower mortality rate may be caused by the widespread use of ICDs in this population (>80%) but highlights that these patients are at high risk for morbidity with recurrent ICD shocks. In series documenting outcomes after ablation the rates of recurrence after ablation range from 18% to 60% within 6 months requiring a second procedure; after second ablation all studies reported no recurrence.[25,26,31]

SUMMARY

PVCs, although generally considered benign, have been associated with increased morbidity and mortality. Patients with structurally normal hearts and frequent PVCs should be offered complete work-up to exclude structural heart disease and if they remain asymptomatic should be followed closely with at least annual evaluation and echocardiography to screen for PVC induced cardiomyopathy. Both catheter ablation and medical therapy have been shown to reduce the burden and potentially improve the EF in patients with PVC-induced cardiomyopathy. PVC-induced VF is a malignant variety of PVC for which the mechanism is incompletely elucidated; however, catheter ablation may reduce ICD shocks.

REFERENCES

1. Hiss RG, Lamb LE. Electrocardiographic findings in 122,043 individuals. Circulation 1962;25:947–61.
2. Jouven X, Zureik M, Desnos M, et al. Long-term outcome in asymptomatic men with exercise-induced premature ventricular depolarizations. N Engl J Med 2000;343(12):826–33.
3. Hingorani P, Karnad DR, Rohekar P, et al. Arrhythmias seen in baseline 24-hour holter ECG recordings in healthy normal volunteers during phase 1 clinical trials. Journal of Clinical Pharma 2016. [Epub ahead of print].
4. Kennedy HL, Whitlock JA, Sprague MK, et al. Long-term follow-up of asymptomatic healthy subjects with frequent and complex ventricular ectopy. N Engl J Med 1985;312(4):193–7.
5. Simpson RJ Jr, Cascio WE, Schreiner PJ, et al. Prevalence of premature ventricular contractions in a population of African American and white men and women: the Atherosclerosis Risk in Communities (ARIC) study. Am Heart J 2002;143(3):535–40.
6. Glasser SP, Clark PI, Applebaum HJ. Occurrence of frequent complex arrhythmias detected by ambulatory monitoring: findings in an apparently healthy asymptomatic elderly population. Chest 1979; 75(5):565–8.
7. Crow RS, Prineas RJ, Dias V, et al. Ventricular premature beats in a population sample. frequency and associations with coronary risk characteristics. Circulation 1975;52(Suppl 6):III211–5.
8. Iwai S, Cantillon DJ, Kim RJ, et al. Right and left ventricular outflow tract tachycardias: evidence for a common electrophysiologic mechanism. J Cardiovasc Electrophysiol 2006;17(10):1052–8.
9. Lerman BB, Belardinelli L, West GA, et al. Adenosine-sensitive ventricular tachycardia: evidence suggesting cyclic AMP-mediated triggered activity. Circulation 1986;74(2):270–80.
10. Lerman BB, Stein K, Engelstein ED, et al. Mechanism of repetitive monomorphic ventricular tachycardia. Circulation 1995;92(3):421–9.
11. Crawford T, Mueller G, Sarsam S, et al. Magnetic resonance imaging for identifying patients with cardiac sarcoidosis and preserved or mildly reduced left ventricular function at risk of ventricular arrhythmias. Circ Arrhythm Electrophysiol 2014;7(6): 1109–15.
12. Marcus FI, Zareba W, Calkins H, et al. Arrhythmogenic right ventricular cardiomyopathy/dysplasia clinical presentation and diagnostic evaluation: results from the North American multidisciplinary study. Heart Rhythm 2009;6(7):984–92.
13. Casella M, Pizzamiglio F, Dello Russo A, et al. Feasibility of combined unipolar and bipolar voltage maps to improve sensitivity of endomyocardial biopsy. Circ Arrhythm Electrophysiol 2015;8(3):625–32.
14. Riley MP, Zado E, Bala R, et al. Lack of uniform progression of endocardial scar in patients with arrhythmogenic right ventricular dysplasia/cardiomyopathy and ventricular tachycardia. Circ Arrhythm Electrophysiol 2010;3(4):332–8.
15. Campos B, Jauregui ME, Park KM, et al. New unipolar electrogram criteria to identify irreversibility of nonischemic left ventricular cardiomyopathy. J Am Coll Cardiol 2012;60(21):2194–204.
16. Santangeli P, Hamilton-Craig C, Dello Russo A, et al. Imaging of scar in patients with ventricular arrhythmias of right ventricular origin: cardiac magnetic resonance versus electroanatomic mapping. J Cardiovasc Electrophysiol 2011;22(12):1359–66.
17. Bikkina M, Larson MG, Levy D. Prognostic implications of asymptomatic ventricular arrhythmias: the Framingham Heart Study. Ann Intern Med 1992; 117(12):990–6.
18. Abdalla IS, Prineas RJ, Neaton JD, et al. Relation between ventricular premature complexes and sudden cardiac death in apparently healthy men. Am J Cardiol 1987;60(13):1036–42.
19. Ataklte F, Erqou S, Laukkanen J, et al. Meta-analysis of ventricular premature complexes and their relation to cardiac mortality in general populations. Am J Cardiol 2013;112(8):1263–70.
20. Dukes JW, Dewland TA, Vittinghoff E, et al. Ventricular ectopy as a predictor of heart failure and death. J Am Coll Cardiol 2015;66(2):101–9.
21. Lin CY, Chang SL, Lin YJ, et al. Long-term outcome of multiform premature ventricular complexes

in structurally normal heart. Int J Cardiol 2015;180: 80–5.

22. Agarwal SK, Chao J, Peace F, et al. Premature ventricular complexes on screening electrocardiogram and risk of ischemic stroke. Stroke 2015;46(5): 1365–7.

23. Haissaguerre M, Shoda M, Jais P, et al. Mapping and ablation of idiopathic ventricular fibrillation. Circulation 2002;106(8):962–7.

24. Nogami A, Sugiyasu A, Kubota S, et al. Mapping and ablation of idiopathic ventricular fibrillation from the purkinje system. Heart Rhythm 2005;2(6): 646–9.

25. Knecht S, Sacher F, Wright M, et al. Long-term follow-up of idiopathic ventricular fibrillation ablation: a multi-center study. J Am Coll Cardiol 2009;54(6):522–8.

26. Van Herendael H, Zado ES, Haqqani H, et al. Catheter ablation of ventricular fibrillation: importance of left ventricular outflow tract and papillary muscle triggers. Heart Rhythm 2014;11(4):566–73.

27. Haissaguerre M, Shah DC, Jais P, et al. Role of purkinje conducting system in triggering of idiopathic ventricular fibrillation. Lancet 2002; 359(9307):677–8.

28. Haissaguerre M, Derval N, Sacher F, et al. Sudden cardiac arrest associated with early repolarization. N Engl J Med 2008;358(19):2016–23.

29. Srivathsan K, Gami AS, Ackerman MJ, et al. Treatment of ventricular fibrillation in a patient with prior diagnosis of long QT syndrome: importance of precise electrophysiologic diagnosis to successfully ablate the trigger. Heart Rhythm 2007;4(8):1090–3.

30. Pasquie JL, Sanders P, Hocini M, et al. Fever as a precipitant of idiopathic ventricular fibrillation in patients with normal hearts. J Cardiovasc Electrophysiol 2004;15(11):1271–6.

31. Sadek MM, Benhayon D, Sureddi R, et al. Idiopathic ventricular arrhythmias originating from the moderator band: electrocardiographic characteristics and treatment by catheter ablation. Heart Rhythm 2015;12(1):67–75.

32. Derval N, Simpson CS, Birnie DH, et al. Prevalence and characteristics of early repolarization in the CASPER registry: cardiac arrest survivors with preserved ejection fraction registry. J Am Coll Cardiol 2011;58(7):722–8.

33. Survivors of out-of-hospital cardiac arrest with apparently normal heart need for definition and standardized clinical evaluation. Consensus statement of the joint steering committees of the unexplained cardiac arrest registry of Europe and of the idiopathic ventricular fibrillation registry of the United States. Circulation 1997;95(1):265–72.

34. Li P, Rudy Y. A model of canine Purkinje cell electrophysiology and ca(2+) cycling: rate dependence, triggered activity, and comparison to ventricular myocytes. Circ Res 2011;109(1):71–9.

35. Antzelevitch C, Sicouri S. Clinical relevance of cardiac arrhythmias generated by afterdepolarizations role of M cells in the generation of U waves, triggered activity and torsade de pointes. J Am Coll Cardiol 1994;23(1):259–77.

36. Kamkin A, Kiseleva I, Isenberg G. Stretch-activated currents in ventricular myocytes: amplitude and arrhythmogenic effects increase with hypertrophy. Cardiovasc Res 2000;48(3):409–20.

37. Hansen DE, Craig CS, Hondeghem LM. Stretch-induced arrhythmias in the isolated canine ventricle. evidence for the importance of mechanoelectrical feedback. Circulation 1990;81(3):1094–105.

38. He B, Lu Z, He W, et al. The effects of atrial ganglionated plexi stimulation on ventricular electrophysiology in a normal canine heart. J Interv Card Electrophysiol 2013;37(1):1–8.

39. Deo M, Boyle PM, Kim AM, et al. Arrhythmogenesis by single ectopic beats originating in the Purkinje system. Am J Physiol Heart Circ Physiol 2010; 299(4):H1002–11.

40. Cooper MW. Postextrasystolic potentiation. do we really know what it means and how to use it? Circulation 1993;88(6):2962–71.

41. Wichterle D, Melenovsky V, Simek J, et al. Hemodynamics and autonomic control of heart rate turbulence. J Cardiovasc Electrophysiol 2006;17(3):286–91.

42. Segerson NM, Wasmund SL, Abedin M, et al. Heart rate turbulence parameters correlate with post-premature ventricular contraction changes in muscle sympathetic activity. Heart Rhythm 2007;4(3): 284–9.

43. Spragg DD, Kass DA. Pathobiology of left ventricular dyssynchrony and resynchronization. Prog Cardiovasc Dis 2006;49(1):26–41.

44. Wijnmaalen AP, Delgado V, Schalij MJ, et al. Beneficial effects of catheter ablation on left ventricular and right ventricular function in patients with frequent premature ventricular contractions and preserved ejection fraction. Heart 2010;96(16): 1275–80.

45. Hasdemir C, Ulucan C, Yavuzgil O, et al. Tachycardia-induced cardiomyopathy in patients with idiopathic ventricular arrhythmias: the incidence, clinical and electrophysiologic characteristics, and the predictors. J Cardiovasc Electrophysiol 2011; 22(6):663–8.

46. Baman TS, Lange DC, Ilg KJ, et al. Relationship between burden of premature ventricular complexes and left ventricular function. Heart Rhythm 2010; 7(7):865–9.

47. Ban JE, Park HC, Park JS, et al. Electrocardiographic and electrophysiological characteristics of premature ventricular complexes associated with left ventricular dysfunction in patients without structural heart disease. Europace 2013;15(5): 735–41.

48. Niwano S, Wakisaka Y, Niwano H, et al. Prognostic significance of frequent premature ventricular contractions originating from the ventricular outflow tract in patients with normal left ventricular function. Heart 2009;95(15):1230–7.

49. Carballeira Pol L, Deyell MW, Frankel DS, et al. Ventricular premature depolarization QRS duration as a new marker of risk for the development of ventricular premature depolarization-induced cardiomyopathy. Heart Rhythm 2014;11(2):299–306.

50. Bogun F, Crawford T, Reich S, et al. Radiofrequency ablation of frequent, idiopathic premature ventricular complexes: comparison with a control group without intervention. Heart Rhythm 2007;4(7):863–7.

51. Sadron Blaye-Felice M, Hamon D, Sacher F, et al. Premature ventricular contraction-induced cardiomyopathy: related clinical and electrophysiologic parameters. Heart Rhythm 2015;13(1):103–10.

52. Lu F, Benditt DG, Yu J, et al. Effects of catheter ablation of "asymptomatic" frequent ventricular premature complexes in patients with reduced (<48%) left ventricular ejection fraction. Am J Cardiol 2012;110(6):852–6.

53. Del Carpio Munoz F, Syed FF, Noheria A, et al. Characteristics of premature ventricular complexes as correlates of reduced left ventricular systolic function: study of the burden, duration, coupling interval, morphology and site of origin of PVCs. J Cardiovasc Electrophysiol 2011;22(7):791–8.

54. Yokokawa M, Kim HM, Good E, et al. Relation of symptoms and symptom duration to premature ventricular complex-induced cardiomyopathy. Heart Rhythm 2012;9(1):92–5.

55. Yokokawa M, Kim HM, Good E, et al. Impact of QRS duration of frequent premature ventricular complexes on the development of cardiomyopathy. Heart Rhythm 2012;9(9):1460–4.

56. Yokokawa M, Good E, Crawford T, et al. Recovery from left ventricular dysfunction after ablation of frequent premature ventricular complexes. Heart Rhythm 2013;10(2):172–5.

57. Deyell MW, Park KM, Han Y, et al. Predictors of recovery of left ventricular dysfunction after ablation of frequent premature ventricular depolarizations. Heart Rhythm 2012;9(9):1465–72.

58. Mountantonakis SE, Frankel DS, Gerstenfeld EP, et al. Reversal of outflow tract ventricular premature depolarization-induced cardiomyopathy with ablation: effect of residual arrhythmia burden and preexisting cardiomyopathy on outcome. Heart Rhythm 2011;8(10):1608–14.

59. European Heart Rhythm Association, Heart Rhythm Society, Zipes DP, Camm AJ, Borggrefe M, et al. ACC/AHA/ESC 2006 guidelines for management of patients with ventricular arrhythmias and the prevention of sudden cardiac death: a report of the American College of Cardiology/American Heart Association task force and the European Society of Cardiology committee for practice guidelines (writing committee to develop guidelines for management of patients with ventricular arrhythmias and the prevention of sudden cardiac death). J Am Coll Cardiol 2006;48(5):e247–346.

60. Krittayaphong R, Bhuripanyo K, Punlee K, et al. Effect of atenolol on symptomatic ventricular arrhythmia without structural heart disease: a randomized placebo-controlled study. Am Heart J 2002;144(6):e10.

61. Withagen AJ, Corbeij HM, Huige MC, et al. Effects of epanolol and metoprolol on the heart measured by 24-hour Holter monitoring. Drugs 1989;38(Suppl 2):67–9.

62. Capucci A, Di Pasquale G, Boriani G, et al. A double-blind crossover comparison of flecainide and slow-release mexiletine in the treatment of stable premature ventricular complexes. Int J Clin Pharmacol Res 1991;11(1):23–33.

63. Echt DS, Liebson PR, Mitchell LB, et al. Mortality and morbidity in patients receiving encainide, flecainide, or placebo. The Cardiac Arrhythmia Suppression Trial. N Engl J Med 1991;324(12):781–8.

64. Hohnloser SH, Meinertz T, Stubbs P, et al. Efficacy and safety of d-sotalol, a pure class III antiarrhythmic compound, in patients with symptomatic complex ventricular ectopy. Results of a multicenter, randomized, double-blind, placebo-controlled dose-finding study. The d-Sotalol PVC Study Group. Circulation 1995;92(6):1517–25.

65. Lidell C, Rehnqvist N, Sjogren A, et al. Comparative efficacy of oral sotalol and procainamide in patients with chronic ventricular arrhythmias: a multicenter study. Am Heart J 1985;109(5 Pt 1):970–5.

66. Kubac G, Klinke WP, Grace M. Randomized double blind trial comparing sotalol and propranolol in chronic ventricular arrhythmia. Can J Cardiol 1988;4(7):355–9.

67. Singh SN, Fletcher RD, Fisher SG, et al. Amiodarone in patients with congestive heart failure and asymptomatic ventricular arrhythmia. survival trial of antiarrhythmic therapy in congestive heart failure. N Engl J Med 1995;333(2):77–82.

68. Betensky BP, Park RE, Marchlinski FE, et al. The V(2) transition ratio: a new electrocardiographic criterion for distinguishing left from right ventricular outflow tract tachycardia origin. J Am Coll Cardiol 2011;57(22):2255–62.

69. Bogun F, Taj M, Ting M, et al. Spatial resolution of pace mapping of idiopathic ventricular tachycardia/ectopy originating in the right ventricular outflow tract. Heart Rhythm 2008;5(3):339–44.

70. Azegami K, Wilber DJ, Arruda M, et al. Spatial resolution of pacemapping and activation mapping in patients with idiopathic right ventricular outflow tract

tachycardia. J Cardiovasc Electrophysiol 2005; 16(8):823–9.

71. Latchamsetty R, Yokokawa M, Morady F, et al. Multicenter outcomes for catheter ablation of idiopathic premature ventricular complexes. J Am Coll Cardiol 2015;1(3):116–23.

72. Takemoto M, Yoshimura H, Ohba Y, et al. Radiofrequency catheter ablation of premature ventricular complexes from right ventricular outflow tract improves left ventricular dilation and clinical status in patients without structural heart disease. J Am Coll Cardiol 2005;45(8):1259–65.

73. Ling Z, Liu Z, Su L, et al. Radiofrequency ablation versus antiarrhythmic medication for treatment of ventricular premature beats from the right ventricular outflow tract: prospective randomized study. Circ Arrhythm Electrophysiol 2014;7(2):237–43.

74. Yarlagadda RK, Iwai S, Stein KM, et al. Reversal of cardiomyopathy in patients with repetitive monomorphic ventricular ectopy originating from the right ventricular outflow tract. Circulation 2005;112(8): 1092–7.

75. Zhong L, Lee YH, Huang XM, et al. Relative efficacy of catheter ablation vs antiarrhythmic drugs in treating premature ventricular contractions: a single-center retrospective study. Heart Rhythm 2014;11(2):187–93.

76. Penela D, Acosta J, Aguinaga L, et al. Ablation of frequent PVC in patients meeting criteria for primary prevention ICD implant: safety of withholding the implant. Heart Rhythm 2015;12(12):2434–42.

77. Ozaydin M, Moazzami K, Kalantarian S, et al. Long-term outcome of patients with idiopathic ventricular fibrillation: a meta-analysis. J Cardiovasc Electrophysiol 2015;26(10):1095–104.

Role of Genetic Testing in Patients with Ventricular Arrhythmias in Apparently Normal Hearts

Nynke Hofman, PhD[a], Arthur A.M. Wilde, MD, PhD[b],*

KEYWORDS

- Ventricular arrhythmias • Sudden cardiac death • Genes • LQTS • CPVT • Brugada syndrome
- SQTS • ERS

KEY POINTS

- It is important to perform cardiological investigations in family members who have died suddenly, and also when there is a negative autopsy.
- Ventricular arrhythmias without structural heart disease are responsible for ~35% of patients who have a sudden cardiac death before the age of 40 years.
- It is important to isolate the DNA of persons who have died suddenly to confirm a (later diagnosed) familial arrhythmia.
- When a pathogenic (causal) mutation is identified in the proband, predictive testing of family members can be offered, leading to timely treatment of identified affected (presymptomatic) individuals.

INTRODUCTION

Ventricular arrhythmias are a major cause of death and usually occur in patients with structural heart disease. Ventricular arrhythmias without structural heart disease are a rare but potentially life-threatening symptom in young patients. Molecular autopsies and/or cardiological investigation of family members have revealed that the primary electrical diseases (ie, the channelopathies) underlie up to 35% of these sudden deaths[1–3] in individuals 1 to 40 years old and up to 70% in infants.[4] During the last 20 years an important part of the molecular basis of the ion channelopathies, including long QT syndrome (LQTS), Brugada syndrome (BrS), catecholaminergic polymorphic ventricular tachycardia (CPVT), and short QT syndrome (SQTS), has to a large extend been identified. Increased knowledge of the genetic basis of the disease sometimes leads to gene-specific treatment in known or suspected disease carriers. From the start it has been proposed that intensive collaboration between cardiologists, clinical geneticists or genetic counselors, and molecular geneticists is warranted for the most accurate patient care as well as research purposes.

Molecular genetic testing usually starts with the proband (the first person in a family who presents with symptoms of a suspected inherited disorder). Molecular testing was for many years targeted to the most likely gene involved (most likely based on the patient/family history and clinical parameters; eg, the morphology of the ST-T segments and the result of the exercise test). With the development of next-generation sequencing (NGS) technology the approach of genetic testing for

[a] Department of Clinical Genetics, Academic Medical Center, M0-229, Meibergdreef 9, Amsterdam 1105 AZ, The Netherlands; [b] Department of Cardiology, Academic Medical Center, B2-239, Meibergdreef 9, Amsterdam 1105 AZ, The Netherlands
* Corresponding author.
E-mail address: a.a.wilde@amc.nl

Card Electrophysiol Clin 8 (2016) 515–523
http://dx.doi.org/10.1016/j.ccep.2016.04.002
1877-9182/16/$ – see front matter © 2016 Elsevier Inc. All rights reserved.

cardiac channelopathies has changed substantially. Extended gene panels can be screened in a short period of time at a low cost. When a pathogenic (causal) mutation is identified in the proband, predictive testing of family members can be offered, leading to timely treatment of identified affected (presymptomatic) individuals. For the inherited arrhythmia syndromes it has been shown that during a follow-up of 3 to 4 years prophylactic treatment was installed in up to 70% to 80% of presymptomatically tested patients with LQTS and CPVT.[5] Besides the identification of a pathogenic mutation, in the past few years research has revealed the importance of genetic variants that (potentially) modify the clinical phenotype (ie, genetic modifiers). These variants have direct or indirect effects; for example, by modifying protein expression on the severity of the phenotype. This article reviews the current molecular understanding of the primary electrical diseases of the heart that are associated with sudden cardiac death, and provides a summary of the causal genes (**Table 1**).

THE MECHANISM OF ELECTROPHYSIOLOGY AND ELECTROPHYSIOLOGIC ABNORMALITIES

Ion channels are transmembrane proteins that conduct ions through the cell membrane. They provide the cellular basis for cardiac electrical activity. The channels have specific ion selectivity and are responsible for timely regulation of the passage of charged ions across the cell membrane in myocytes (the process of depolarization and repolarization). Depolarization is caused by an inward current of positively charged ions (ie, sodium and calcium ions) into the cell. Repolarization is caused by potassium and calcium channels (outward current of, respectively, K^+ and Ca^{2+} ions). Impairment in the flow of ions in and out of heart cells leads to a disturbance of the cardiac action potential morphology and provides a substrate for cardiac arrhythmias. This aberrant behavior of ion channels can be caused by pathogenic mutations in the genes that encode for these proteins.

MOLECULAR GENETICS OF LONG QT SYNDROME

LQTS is an inherited arrhythmia syndrome, characterized by an abnormally prolonged QT interval and abnormal T-wave morphology leading to life-threatening arrhythmias and sudden cardiac death. Jervell and Lange-Nielsen[6] first described LQTS in 1957. They reported a family with a

prolonged QT interval and congenital deafness, many years later shown to be caused by a homozygous KCNQ1 mutation. The disorder, now known as the very rare Jervell and Lange-Nielsen syndrome, is inherited as an autosomal recessive trait. In 1963 and 1964 respectively Romano and colleagues[7] and Ward[8] described families presenting with QT prolongation, recurrent syncope, and sudden death, without deafness and transmitted as an autosomal dominant trait. Based on a population study, the prevalence of LQTS is now estimated as being as high as 1 in 2000.[9]

The diagnosis is made on the patient's history (episodic dizziness, syncope, palpitations, triggers of [near] syncope and family history), and by abnormal QT-interval prolongation on the electrocardiogram (ECG). The symptoms may be confused with epilepsy.[10] In 2010 Viskin and colleagues[11] described that patients with LQTS have an insufficient QT-interval shortening in response to the mild abrupt tachycardia provoked by standing up from a supine position, which can easily be used as a noninvasive bedside test to reach the diagnosis. Alternatively, the response of the QTc interval during exercise, and in particular during the recovery phase of an exercise test, is abnormal for the most important LQT subtypes.[12]

The values of the QTc (rate corrected using the Bazett formula) differ slightly between men and women and are age specific. The risk of cardiac events is higher in boys until the teenage years, but higher in women during adulthood.[13–16]

The Role of Genetic Testing in Long QT Syndrome

Mutations in at least 15 genes have been reported (see **Table 1**).

Genetic testing reveals a mutation in 60% to 75% of patients with a clear phenotype, and this proportion is even higher in familial cases.[17–20] LQT1, LQT2, and LQT3, named in chronologic order of identification, are by far the most commonly found genotypes, accounting for at least 85% of the genotyped LQTS.[21] In these most common subtypes there is a clear phenotype-genotype correlation: syncope and sudden death are most commonly triggered by exercise and swimming in KCNQ1 mutations (LQT1) and occur mostly at rest with SCN5A mutations (LQT3). Arrhythmias in LQT2, with mutations in KCNH2, are often triggered by acoustic stimuli (alarm clocks, telephones) and stress.[22,23] Female LQT2 carriers should receive extra monitoring in the months after delivery, because this period has been identified as a period of increased risk, possibly because of the combined effects of hormonal imbalance, stress, and fatigue.[24,25] The choice of treatment is mostly based on the underlying gene defect, so genetic testing is important to determine optimal treatment strategies.[25] Furthermore, all carriers should receive gene-specific lifestyle modification instructions and a list of drugs that must be avoided because they may precipitate lethal arrhythmias (www.qtdrugs.org). However, some lifestyle adaptions are gene specific; they relate in particular to the gene-specific triggers (discussed earlier). In family members, genetic testing of the familial mutation is important because of the variable expression and penetrance of the disease; a normal QTc value does not rule out carriership.[26] A prolonged QT value can be acquired as a result of side effects from medications or metabolic disease.[27] It is estimated that, in these cases of acquired LQTS, approximately 15% of cases is based on a (concealed) pathogenic mutation in one of the LQT genes.[28,29]

BRUGADA SYNDROME

It has been postulated that also BrS is also a primary electrical disease. It is characterized by right ventricular conduction delay and ST elevation in the right precordial ECG leads and was first described in 1992.[30] However, in more recent years it has been postulated that BrS is a predominant right ventricular outflow tract disease with local fibrosis, which leads to systematic discrete abnormal MRI findings.[31–33] It is associated with syncope and premature sudden death caused by ventricular fibrillation (VF). Arrhythmias are often induced by fever and predominantly occur at rest or during sleep. The disease has an age-related and sex-related penetrance; most arrhythmic events occur in men in and around the fourth decade of life.[34] BrS can only be diagnosed in the presence of a type I ECG pattern; that is, a coved ST-segment elevation greater than or equal to 0.2 mV, in more than 1 precordial lead positioned in the second, third, or fourth intercostal space, occurring spontaneously or after a provocative drug test with intravenous administration of class I antiarrhythmic drugs.[35] The prevalence of a BrS-type ECG has been estimated between 1 in 2000 and 1 in 5000.[36]

The Role of Genetic Testing in Brugada Syndrome

Loss-of-function mutations in the cardiac sodium channel subunit, SCN5A, have been identified in 25% to 30% of patients with Brugada, most of which are dominant missense mutations with loss-of-function characteristics. Other possible disease-causing genes have been described (see **Table 1**), but do not reveal many causal mutations. A mutation analysis of 12 known BrS-susceptibility genes in a large cohort of unrelated patients with BrS identified SCN5A mutations in 16%, with the other 11 genes accounting for less than 5% of patients.[37] In recent years it has been postulated that the genetic basis of BrS might be oligogenic (ie, caused by a small number of genetic variants).[38] Various studies have indicated that asymptomatic carriers with a normal baseline ECG are at low risk for arrhythmias. All mutation carriers receive a list of drugs that must be avoided (www.brugadadrugs.org)[39] and should be instructed to obtain an ECG in case of fever (temperature ≥38.5°C) at least once to assess whether their form of BrS is hyperthermia sensitive or at least use antipyretic drugs to reduce the temperature. Symptomatic patients should be treated with an implantable cardioverter-defibrillator (ICD) and the treatment of asymptomatic patients is a matter of dispute.[40]

Because there is no clear genotype-phenotype relationship, the role for genetic testing in BrS is less clear than in LQTS. More importantly, a negative baseline phenotype in members of families with a putative SCN5A mutation does not disclose the presence of a phenotype in genotype-negative family members.[41] This finding effectively means that in these families clinicians cannot limit the familial evaluation to genetic testing only.

CATECHOLAMINERGIC POLYMORPHIC VENTRICULAR TACHYCARDIA

CPVT was first described in a case report of 3 affected sisters in 1960, although it was described as multifocal ventricular extrasystoles, and not yet as CPVT.[42] In 1975 Reid and colleagues[43] described a bidirectional VT precipitated by effort and emotional stress in a 6-year-old girl with no evidence of structural heart disease who survived a cardiac arrest. The first larger series of patients with CPVT (with follow-up) was described by Leenhardt and colleagues[44] in 1995. CPVT is an inherited, exercise induced arrhythmia in a structurally normal heart. Symptoms can already occur at young, preschool age. Typical for CPVT is the normal baseline ECG, although bradycardia is frequently observed. Polymorphic VT's are unmasked during exercise testing in most affected patients.[45] Treatment mainly consists of β-blocker therapy and is effective in most patients, although not all ectopy disappears during therapy. In those cases in which β-blockers are not sufficiently protective, flecainide can be added, and, when the combined pharmacologic treatment is not

Table 1
Genetic basis of the inherited arrhythmia syndromes

Disease	Subtype	Chromosomal Locus	Mode of Transmission	Gene	Ion Current Affected	Effect	Protein
LQTS	LQT1	11p15.5	AD/AR	KCNQ1	IKs	↓	KvLQT1
	LQT2	7q35-q36	AD	KCNH2	IKr	↓	HERG
	LQT3	3P21	AD	SCN5A	INa	↑	Nav1.5
	LQT4	4q25-q27	AD	ANK2	Decreased coordination of Ncx, Na/K ATPase	—	Ankyrin-B
	LQT5	21q22.1-q22.2	AD/AR	KCNE1	IKs	↓	minK
	LQT6	21q22.1	AD	KCNE2	IKr	↓	MiRP1
	LQT7	17q23.1-24.2	AD	KCNJ2	IK1	↓	Kir2.1
	LQT8	12p13.3	AD	CACNA1C	ICa-L	↑	Cav1.2
	LQT9	3p25	AD	CAV3	Ina	↑	Caveolin-3
	LQT10	11q23	AD	SCN4B	Ina	↑	Navβ4
	LQT11	7q21-q22	AD	AKAP9	IKs	↓	Yotiao
	LQT12	20q11.2	AD	SNTA1	Ina	↑	1-syntrophin
	LQT13	11q24	AD	KCNJ5	Ik1	↓	Kir3.4
	LQT14	14q32.11	AD	CALM1	Dysfunctional Ca^{2+} signaling	—	Calmodulin
	LQT15	2p21	AD	CALM2	Dysfunctional Ca^{2+} signaling	—	Calmodulin
BrS	BrS1	3p21	AD	SCN5A	Ina	↓	Nav1.5
	BrS2	3p24	AD	GPD1L	Ina	↓	GPD1-L
	BrS3	12p13.3	AD	CACNA1C	ICa-L	↓	Cav1.2
	BrS4	10p12.33	AD	CACNB2B	ICa-L	↓	Cavβ2b
	BrS5	19q13.1	AD	SCN1B	Ina	↓	Navβ.1
	BrS6	11q13-q14	AD	KCNE3	IKs/ITo	↑	MiRP2
	BrS7	11q23.3	AD	SCN3B	Ina	↓	Navβ.3
	BrS8	12p11.23	AD	KCNJ8	Ik-ATP	↑	Kir6.1
	BrS9	15q24.1	AD	HCN4	—	—	Hyperpolarization cyclic nucleotide-gated 4
	BrS10	17p13.1	AD	RANGRF	Ina	↓	RAN-G release factor (MOG1)
	BrS11	Xq23	AD	KCNE5	—	—	Potassium voltage-gated channel subfamily E member 1-like
	Brs12	1p13.2	AD	KCND3	Ito	↑	Kv4.3
	Brs13	7q21.11	AD	CACNA2D1	Ica	↓	Cavα2d
	BrS14	3p14.3	AD	SLMAP	—	—	Sarcolemma-associated protein
	BrS15	19q13.33	AD	TRPM4	—	—	Transient receptor potential M4
	BrS16	11q23.3	AD	SCN2B	Ina	↓	Navβ2
	BrS17	3p22.2	AD	SCN10A	—	—	Navβ
	BrS18	12p12.1	AD	ABCC9	Ik-ATP	↑	Sur2A
	BrS19	12p11.21	AD	PKP2	—	—	Plakophilin-2

CPVT	CPVT1	1q42.1-q43	AD	RYR2	SR Ca²⁺ release	Ryanodine receptor	↑
	CPVT2	1p13.3-p11	AR	CASQ2	SR Ca²⁺ release	Calsequestrin	↑
	CPVT3	17q23.1–24.2	AD	KCNJ2	IK1	Kir2.1	→
	CPVT4	6q22-q23	AR	TRDN	SR Ca²⁺ release	Tradin	→
	CPVT5	14q31-q32	AD	CALM1	SR Ca²⁺ release	Calmodulin	→
SQTS	SQT1	7q35-q36	AD	KCNH2	IKr	HERG	↑
	SQT2	11p15.5	AD	KCNQ1	IKs	KvLQT1	↑
	SQT3	17q23.1–24.2	AD	KCNJ2	IK1	Kir2.1	↑
ERS	ERS1	12p11.23	AD	KCNJ8	IK-ATP	Kir 6.1	↑
	ERS2	12p13.3	AD	CACNa1C	Ica	Cav1.2	→
	ERS3	10p12.33	AD	CACNB2b	Ica	Cavβ2b	→
	ERS4	7q21.11	AD	CACNA2D1	Ica	Cavα2d	→
	ERS5	12p12.1	AD	ABCC9	Ik-ATP	SUR2A	↑
	ERS6	3p21	AD	SCN5A	Ina	Nav1.5	→
	ERS7?	7q31.31	AD	KCND2	—	Perrin Mj et al 2014	—

Abbreviations: AD, autosomal dominant; AR, autosomal recessive.

sufficiently effective, ablation of the left ganglion stellatum is a good option.[35,46]

The Role of Genetic Testing in Catecholaminergic Polymorphic Ventricular Tachycardia

In approximately 60% of patients with CPVT a pathogenic mutation is found in the RYR2 gene.[47–49] The phenotype within families is variable and nonpenetrance can be observed.[45] In families with an autosomal recessive pattern of inheritance, CASQ2 mutations have been identified.[50,51] Homozygous CASQ2-mutation carriers are affected by a severe phenotype, whereas heterozygous carriers often are asymptomatic or mildly affected. More recently, the CALM1 and TRDN genes have been implicated as a cause for CPVT in a linkage and a candidate gene approach respectively.[52,53]

It is generally accepted to start treatment in all carriers of a pathogenic RyR2 mutation.[35] The presence of incomplete penetrance effectively means that all family members of a RyR2 proband should be genotyped. Also, lifestyle advice is pertinent for all carriers of a pathogenic RyR2 mutation: limiting/avoiding competitive sports, limiting/avoiding strenuous exercise, and limiting stressful environments.

SHORT QT SYNDROME

SQTS is a rare inherited channelopathy, characterized by a shortened QTc interval on the ECG (<330 milliseconds), syncope, paroxysmal atrial fibrillation, and cardiac arrhythmias.[54,55] Mutations have been identified in genes encoding for the potassium channels KCNH2, KCNQ1, and KCNJ2. Mutations in calcium channel subunits (CACNA1C, CACNB2) are associated with BrS with shorter than normal QTc intervals.[56] The yield of genetic testing in SQTS is low; in a recent study of 45 probands with SQTS, genetic testing revealed a mutation in only 14%.[57] Family members of carriers of a pathogenic mutation probably should be genotyped, but only in combination with the phenotype prophylactic treatment should be installed.[35]

IDIOPATHIC VENTRICULAR FIBRILLATION

Idiopathic VF is defined as spontaneous occurrence of VF in the absence of known causes that may lead to cardiac arrest and therefore remain unexplained. It occurs in families and, because of the lack of phenotype, affected individuals can not be identified before they develop symptoms, which has led to prophylactic ICD implants in whole families. In the Netherlands, a founder haplotype for idiopathic VF was identified in some large families.[58] The haplotype is located on chromosome 7q36 and harbors a large part of the DPP6 gene. DPP6 encodes for a protein that presumably modifies the amplitude of the transient outward current I_{TO}, which is active in the early phase of the action potential. The clinical phenotype is characterized by short-coupled extrasystoles presumably originating from the Purkinje network in the apical anterior part of the right ventricle. It is a malignant disease with, in men, 50% mortality by approximately 55 years of age. The presence of this haplotype, with unknown impact on cardiac function, enables the identification of individuals who are at risk and, importantly, those without risk so that unnecessary ICD implants can be avoided. Hence, in this setting it can be argued that offering genetic testing is of critical importance.

CONDUCTION DISEASE

Cardiac conduction disease is characterized by unexplained progressive cardiac conduction abnormalities and may lead to syncope and sudden death.[59] Most familial cardiac conduction disease in the absence of structural heart disease is caused by mutations in SCN5A.[25,59] Mutations in TRPM4 have been reported in several families with cardiac conduction disease.[60] Sinus node disease has been associated with SCN5A and HCN4 mutations.[61]

EARLY REPOLARIZATION SYNDROME

A subset of idiopathic VF is associated with an ECG characterized by J-point elevation, or early repolarization (ER).[62,63] This category of patients should probably be taken out of the idiopathic VF cohort, because it is becoming clear that ER represents a separate clinical entity. ER is defined as greater than or equal to 1 mm of J-point elevation in at least 2 contiguous ECG leads, with the exception of the right precordial leads (V1–V3) in patients resuscitated from otherwise unexplained VF/polymorphic VT.[37] Almost all individuals with ER syndrome (ERS) are at no or minimal risk for arrhythmic events and sudden cardiac arrest.[64] Incidental discovery of a J wave on routine screening should not be interpreted as a marker of high risk for sudden cardiac death because the odds of this leading to a fatal outcome are low.[65] Candidate gene studies have identified rare variants (in single patients) associated with ERS in 7 genes (see **Table 1**). The role of routine genetic testing in this condition has yet to be proved.

DISCUSSION: HOW TO JUDGE THE VARIANTS

With the development of NGS, large gene panels are readily available and cost-effective. However, besides the increased likelihood of finding a disease-causing mutation, the chance of finding variants of unknown significance also increases. A multidisciplinary team of (genetically) specialized cardiologists, genetic counselors, and molecular geneticists is necessary to judge all the available details of phenotype and genotype to ultimately decide on the significance of the involved variant and family strategies. First it starts with a definite diagnosis in the proband/family. In general, genetic testing should only be used to confirm the diagnosis, not to establish a diagnosis. Once there is a certain pathogenic mutation in the family, it is possible to offer predictive testing of the mutation in relatives (in a genetic counseling process). The mutation carriers should be referred for cardiological investigation and follow-up and the noncarriers can be reassured in most conditions. When there is doubt about the diagnosis, or the significance of the mutation, predictive testing should not be offered, and in this situation all relatives should visit a cardiologist to obtain facts about their own cardiological status.[66,67]

REFERENCES

1. Tan HL, Hofman N, van Langen IM, et al. Sudden unexplained death: heritability and diagnostic yield of cardiological and genetic examination in surviving relatives. Circulation 2005;112:207–13.

2. Tester DJ, Ackerman MJ. Sudden infant death syndrome: how significant are the cardiac channelopathies? Cardiovasc Res 2005;67:388–96.

3. Tester DJ, Ackerman MJ. Postmortem long QT syndrome genetic testing for sudden unexplained death in the young. J Am Coll Cardiol 2007;49:240–6.

4. Van der Werf C, Hofman N, Tan HL, et al. Diagnostic yield in sudden unexplained death and aborted cardiac arrest in the young: the experience of a tertiary referral center in the Netherlands. Heart Rhythm 2010;7:1383–9.

5. Hofman N, Tan HL, Alders M, et al. Active cascade screening in primary inherited arrhythmia syndromes: does it lead to prophylactic treatment? J Am Coll Cardiol 2010;55:2570–6.

6. Jervell A, Lange-Nielsen F. Congenital deaf-mutism, functional heart disease with prolongation of the QT-interval, and sudden death. Am Heart J 1957;54:59–68.

7. Romano C, Gemme G, Pongiglione R. Aritmie cardiache rare dell'eta' pediatrica. Clinica Pediatrica 1963;45:656–83.

8. Ward OC. A new familial cardiac syndrome in children. J Ir Med Assoc 1964;54:103–6.

9. Schwartz PJ, Stramba-Badiale M, Crotti L, et al. Prevalence of the long QT syndrome. Circulation 2009;120:1761–7.

10. Towbin JA, Vatta M. Molecular biology and the prolonged QT syndromes. Am J Med 2001;110:385–98.

11. Viskin S, Postema PG, Bhuiyan ZA, et al. The response of the QT interval to the brief tachycardia provoked by standing: a bedside test for diagnosing long QT syndrome. J Am Coll Cardiol 2010;55:1955–61.

12. Sy RW, van der Werf C, Chattha I, et al. Derivation and validation of a simple exercise-based algorithm for prediction of genetic testing in relatives of LQTS probands. Circulation 2011;124:2187–94.

13. Moss AJ, Robinson JL. Long QT syndrome. Heart Dis Stroke 1992;1:309–14.

14. Rautaharju PM, Zhou SH, Wong S, et al. Sex differences in the evolution of the electrocardiographic QT-interval with age. Can J Cardiol 1992;8:690–5.

15. Locati EH, Zareba W, Moss AJ, et al. Age- and sex-related differences in clinical manifestations in patients with congenital long-QT syndrome: findings from the International LQTS registry. Circulation 1998;97:2237–44.

16. Hobbs JB, Peterson DR, Moss AJ. Risk of aborted cardiac arrest or sudden cardiac death during adolescence in the long-QT syndrome. JAMA 2006;296:1249–54.

17. Splawski I, Shen J, Timothy KW, et al. Spectrum of mutations in long-QT syndrome genes. KVLQT1, HERG, SCN5A, KCNE1 and KCNE2. Circulation 2000;102:1178–85.

18. Kapplinger JD, Tester DJ, Salisbury BA, et al. Spectrum and prevalence of mutations form the first 2,500 consecutive unrelated patients referred for the FAMILION long QT syndrome genetic test. Heart Rhythm 2009;6:1297–303.

19. Kapa S, Tester DJ, Salisbury BA, et al. Genetic testing for long-QT syndrome: distinguishing pathogenic mutations from benign variants. Circulation 2009;120:1752–60.

20. Hofman N, Tan HL, Alders M, et al. Yield of molecular and clinical testing for arrhythmia syndromes, report of a 15 years' experience. Circulation 2013;128:1513–21.

21. Napolitano C, Priori SG, Schwartz PJ, et al. Genetic testing in the long QT syndrome: development and validation of an efficient approach to genotyping in clinical practice. JAMA 2005;294:2975–80.

22. Moss AJ, Robinson JL, Gessman L, et al. Comparison of clinical and genetic variables of cardiac events associated with loud noise versus swimming among subjects with the long QT syndrome. Am J Cardiol 1999;84:876–9.

23. Schwartz PJ. The congenital long QT syndromes from genotype to phenotype: clinical implications. J Intern Med 2006;259:39–47.

24. Seth R, Moss AJ, Mc Nitt S, et al. Long QT syndrome and pregnancy. J Am Coll Cardiol 2007;49:1092–8.

25. Ackerman MJ, Priori SG, Willems S, et al. HRS/EHRA expert consensus statement on the state of genetic testing for the channelopathies and cardiomyopathies. Heart Rhythm 2011;8:1308–39.

26. Hofman N, Wilde AA, Kaab S, et al. Diagnostic criteria for congenital long QT syndrome in the era of molecular genetics. Do we need a scoring system? Eur Heart J 2007;28:575–80.

27. Roden DM, Lazzara R, Rosen M, et al. Multiple mechanisms in the long-QT syndrome. Circulation 1996;94:1996–2012.

28. Williams VS, Cresswell CJ, Ruspi G, et al. Multiplex ligation-dependent probe amplification copy number variant analysis in patients with acquired long QT syndrome. Europace 2015;17:635–41.

29. Itoh H, Crotti L, Aiba T, et al. The genetics underlying acquired long QT syndrome: impact for genetic screening. Eur Heart J 2015. Available at: http://dx.doi.org/10.1093/eurheartj/ehv695.

30. Brugada P, Brugada J. Right bundle branch block, persistent ST elevation and sudden cardiac death: a distinct clinical and electrocardiographic syndrome. J Am Coll Cardiol 1992;20:1391–6.

31. Nademanee K, Raju H, De Noronha S, et al. Fibrosis, connexin 43 and conduction abnormalities in the Brugada syndrome. J Am Coll Cardiol 2015;66:1976–86.

32. van Hoorn F, Campian ME, Spijkerboer A, et al. Mutations in Brugada syndrome are associated with increased cardiac dimensions and reduced contractility. PLoS One 2012;7:e42037.

33. Rudic B, Schimpf R, Veltmann C, et al. Brugada syndrome: clinical presentation and genotype-correlation with magnetic resonance imaging parameters. Europace 2015. Available at: http://dx.doi.org/10.1093/europace/euv300.

34. Antzelevitch C, Brugada P, Borggrefe M, et al. Brugada syndrome: report of the second consensus conference: endorsed by the Heart Rhythm Society and the European Heart Rhythm Association. Circulation 2005;111:659–70.

35. Priori SG, Wilde AA, Horie M, et al. HRS/EHRA/APHRS expert consensus statement on the diagnosis and management of patients with inherited primary arrhythmia syndromes: document endorsed by HRS, EHRA, and APHRS in May 2013 and by ACCF, AHA, PACES, and AEPC in June 2013. Heart Rhythm 2013;10:1932–63.

36. Postema PG. About Brugada syndrome and its prevalence. Europace 2012;14:925–8.

37. Crotti L, Marcou CA, Tester DJ, et al. Spectrum and prevalence of mutations involving BrS1- through BrS12-susceptibility genes in a cohort of unrelated patients referred for Brugada syndrome genetic testing: implications for genetic testing. J Am Coll Cardiol 2012;60:1410–8.

38. Bezzina CR, Barc J, Mizusawa Y, et al. Common variants at SCN5A-SCN10A and HEY2 are associated with Brugada syndrome, a rare disease with high risk of sudden cardiac death. Nat Genet 2013;45:1044–9.

39. Postema PG, Wolpert C, Amin AS, et al. Drugs and Brugada syndrome patients: review of the literature, recommendations, and an up-to-date website (www.brugadadrugs.org). Heart Rhythm 2009;6:1335–41.

40. Mizusawa Y, Wilde AA. Brugada syndrome. Circ Arrhythm Electrophysiol 2012;5:606–16.

41. Probst V, Wilde AAM, Barc J, et al. SCN5A mutations and the role of genetic background in the pathophysiology of Brugada syndrome. Circ Cardiovasc Genet 2009;2:552–7.

42. Berg KJ. Multifocal ventricular extrasystoles with Adams-Stokes syndrome in children. Am Heart J 1960;60:965–70.

43. Reid DS, Tynan M, Braidwood L, et al. Bidirectional tachycardia in a child. A study using His bundle electrography. Br Heart J 1975;37:339–44.

44. Leenhardt A, Lucet V, Denjoy I, et al. Catecholaminergic polymorphic ventricular tachycardia in children. A 7-year follow-up of 21 patients. Circulation 1995;91:1512–9.

45. van der Werf C, Nederend I, Hofman N, et al. Familial evaluation in catecholaminergic polymorphic ventricular tachycardia: disease penetrance and expression in cardiac ryanodine receptor mutation-carrying relatives. Circ Arrhythm Electrophysiol 2012;5:748–56.

46. De Ferrari GM, Dusi V, Spazzolini C, et al. Clinical management of catecholaminergic polymorphic ventricular tachycardia: the role of left cardiac sympathetic denervation. Circulation 2015;131:2185–93.

47. Priori SG, Napolitano C, Tiso N, et al. Mutations in the cardiac ryanodine receptor gene (hRYR2) underlie catecholaminergic polymorphic ventricular tachycardia. Circulation 2001;103:196–200.

48. Laitinen PJ, Brown KM, Piippo K, et al. Mutations of the cardiac ryanodine receptor (hRYR2) gene in familial polymorphic ventricular tachycardia. Circulation 2001;103:485–90.

49. Madeiros-Domingo A, Bhuiyan ZA, Tester DJ, et al. The RYR2-encoded ryanodine receptor/calcium release channel in patients diagnosed previously with either catecholaminergic polymorphic ventricular tachycardia or genotype negative, exercise-induced long QT syndrome: a comprehensive open reading frame mutational analysis. J Am Coll Cardiol 2009;54:2065–74.

50. Lahat H, Pras E, Olender T, et al. A missense mutation in a highly conserved region of CASQ2 is associated with autosomal recessive catecholamine–induced polymorphic ventricular tachycardia in Bedouin families from Israel. Am J Hum Genet 2001;69:1378–84.

51. Postma AV, Denjoy I, Hoorntje TM, et al. Absence of calsequestrin 2 causes severe forms of catecholaminergic polymorphic ventricular tachycardia. Circ Res 2002;91:e21–6.

52. Nyegaard M, Overgaard MT, Sondergaard MT, et al. Mutations in calmodulin cause ventricular tachycardia and sudden cardiac death. Am J Hum Genet 2012;91:703–12.

53. Roux-Buisson N, Cacheux M, Fourest-Lieuvin A, et al. Absence of triadin, a protein of the calcium release complex, is responsible for cardiac arrhythmia with sudden death in human. Hum Mol Genet 2012;21:2759–67.

54. Gussak I, Brugada P, Brugada J, et al. Idiopathic short QT interval: a new clinical syndrome? Cardiology 2000;94:99–102.

55. Gaita F, Giustetto C, Bianchi F, et al. Short QT syndrome: a familial cause of sudden death. Circulation 2003;108:965–70.

56. Antzelevitch C, Pollevick GD, Cordeiro JM, et al. Loss-of-function mutations in the cardiac calcium channel underlie a new clinical entity characterized by ST-segment elevation, short QT intervals, and sudden death. Circulation 2007;115:442–9.

57. Mazzanti A, Kanthan A, Monteforte N, et al. Novel insight into the natural history of short QT syndrome. J Am Coll Cardiol 2014;63:1300–8.

58. Alders M, Koopmann TT, Christaans I, et al. Haplotype-sharing analysis implicates chromosome 7q36 harboring DPP6 in familial idiopathic ventricular fibrillation. Am J Hum Genet 2009;84:468–76.

59. Schott JJ, Alshinawi C, Kyndt F, et al. Cardiac conduction defects associate with mutations in SCN5A. Nat Genet 1999;23:20–1.

60. Kruse M, Schulze-Bahr E, Corfield V, et al. Impaired endocytosis of the ion channel TRPM4 is associated with human progressive familial heart block type 1. J Clin Invest 2009;119:2737–44.

61. Schulze-Bahr E, Neu A, Friederich P, et al. Pacemaker channel dysfunction in a patient with sinus node disease. J Clin Invest 2003;111:1537–45.

62. Rosso R, Kogan E, Belhassen B, et al. J-point elevation in survivors of primary ventricular fibrillation and matched controls subjects: incidence and clinical significance. J Am Coll Cardiol 2008;52:1231–8.

63. Haïssaguerre M, Derval N, Sacher F, et al. Sudden cardiac arrest associated with early repolarization. N Engl J Med 2008;358:2016–23.

64. Antzelevitch C. Genetic, molecular and cellular mechanisms underlying the J-wave syndromes. Circ J 2012;76:1054–65.

65. Rosso R, Adler A, Halkin A, et al. Risk of sudden death among young individuals with J waves and early repolarization: putting the evidence into perspective. Heart Rhythm 2011;8:923–9.

66. Spoonamore KG, Ware SM. Genetic testing and genetic counseling in patients with sudden death risk due to heritable arrhythmias. Heart Rhythm 2016; 13(3):789–97.

67. Ackerman MJ. Genetic purgatory and the cardiac channelopathies: exposing the variants of uncertain/unknown significance issue. Heart Rhythm 2015;12:2325–31.

Nonsustained Ventricular Tachycardia in the Normal Heart
Risk Stratification and Management

 CrossMark

Joseph E. Marine, MD, FHRS

KEYWORDS

- Ventricular tachycardia • Nonsustained • Idiopathic • Risk stratification • Sudden cardiac death
- Antiarrhythmic drug therapy • Catheter ablation • Normal heart

KEY POINTS

- Nonsustained ventricular tachycardia (NSVT) is defined as 3 of more consecutive beats of ventricular origin at a rate of 100 beats/min or greater, lasting less than 30 seconds, usually diagnosed on Holter monitor, telemetry, event recorder, or exercise treadmill test.
- A nonsustained wide-complex tachycardia should be approached in a systematic fashion, considering alternative diagnoses of artifact, paced rhythm, and supraventricular tachycardia with aberrancy, in addition to NSVT.
- Distinction should be made between nonsustained monomorphic and polymorphic ventricular tachycardia, because these entities have distinct differential diagnoses and prognoses.
- A careful approach to exclusion of cardiac ischemia, structural heart disease, and inherited electrical disease should be undertaken before concluding that a patient has a normal heart.
- Treatment options for NSVT in patients with a normal heart without structural or inherited/genetic disease include observation and reassurance; medical therapy with β-blockers, calcium channel blockers, or antiarrhythmic drugs; and ablative therapy. An implantable cardioverter-defibrillator is rarely needed.

INTRODUCTION

Nonsustained ventricular tachycardia (NSVT) is defined as 3 or more consecutive beats of ventricular origin, at a rate of 100 beats per minute (bpm) or greater, lasting less than 30 seconds (**Fig. 1**). NSVT is seen in both the inpatient and outpatient settings, and may be discovered on 12-lead electrocardiogram (ECG), cardiac telemetry, ambulatory ECG monitor, and event monitors. NSVT may also be observed as a finding in patients with cardiac implantable electronic devices, such as pacemakers and insertable loop recorders. NSVT may be symptomatic or asymptomatic; it may be found in otherwise healthy patients as well as those with significant structural heart disease.

Prevalence of NSVT in patients without known heart disease has generally been reported in the range of 0.5% to 1%, and varies with the demographics of the population studied and the intensity of surveillance. In a Framingham Heart Study cohort, NSVT was seen on a single 1-hour ambulatory ECG in 0.53% of 5489 subjects without known coronary heart disease with a mean age of 52.7 years.[1] Hingorani and colleagues[2] reported finding NSVT on 24-hour ambulatory ECG in 0.71% of 1273 healthy volunteers for clinical drug

Conflicts of Interest: None.
Division of Cardiology, Department of Medicine, Johns Hopkins University School of Medicine, 600 North Wolfe Street, Halsted 572, Baltimore, MD 21287, USA
E-mail address: jmarine2@jhmi.edu

Card Electrophysiol Clin 8 (2016) 525–543
http://dx.doi.org/10.1016/j.ccep.2016.04.003
1877-9182/16/$ – see front matter © 2016 Elsevier Inc. All rights reserved.

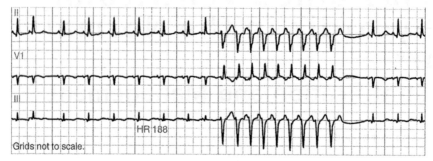

Fig. 1. NSVT discovered on hospital telemetry. A 9-beat run of NSVT at a rate of about 185 bpm is observed on hospital telemetry. The ventricular tachycardia (VT) has a right bundle branch block (RBBB)/superior axis morphology.

studies with a mean age of 41 years. The prevalence of NSVT in older subjects and that found with longer or repeated recordings is likely to be higher.

Regardless of the clinical circumstances, discovery of NSVT frequently triggers concern on the part of the treating physician and patient and leads to consultation directed toward risk stratification and treatment. Because of the association of NSVT with sudden death in patients with significant structural or inherited heart disease, establishing the presence or absence of such disease is a critical component of evaluation of each patient.[3–5] Clinicians should establish a systematic approach to such evaluation.

APPROACH TO EVALUATION OF NONSUSTAINED VENTRICULAR TACHYCARDIA
Overview

In approaching the differential diagnosis of NSVT, a stepwise systematic approach is suggested (**Fig. 2**). First, the consultant should consider that

what may be described as NSVT in a consultation request may not represent a ventricular arrhythmia, and alternative diagnoses should be considered. Second, polymorphic ventricular tachycardia (VT) should be distinguished from monomorphic VT because of substantial differences in differential diagnosis, evaluation, and prognosis. Third, potential causes of VT should be sought, with particular attention paid to determining the presence or absence of structural and/or inherited heart disease, using a focused and targeted evaluation. In addition, a treatment plan should be determined based on degree of symptoms and risk for sudden death. The plan might include medical therapy, catheter ablation, coronary revascularization, implantable cardioverter-defibrillator (ICD) placement, or some combination of these therapies.

Rule out conditions that may mimic ventricular tachycardia
Although wide-complex tachycardia represents VT in most cases in patients with coronary artery

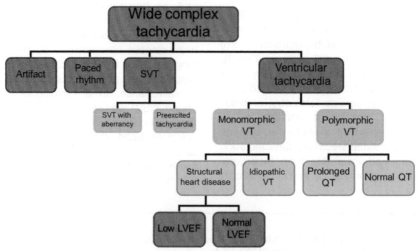

Fig. 2. Stepwise approach to evaluation of NSVT. The diagram outlines a diagnostic approach to a patient presenting with wide-complex tachycardia of undetermined cause. LVEF, left ventricular ejection fraction; SVT, supraventricular tachycardia.

disease (CAD) and congestive heart failure, it is important to consider other possibilities in the differential diagnosis. In particular, the presence of artifact, a paced rhythm, or supraventricular tachycardia (SVT) with conduction aberrancy should be excluded (**Box 1**).

Artifact Artifact is defined as any abnormality seen on telemetry, 12-lead ECG, or ambulatory ECG monitoring that does not reflect a true abnormality of the cardiac rhythm (**Fig. 3**). It is commonly caused by loose monitoring electrodes, mechanical disturbances (tremors, physical motion, and so forth), or electromagnetic interference. To evaluate for ECG artifact, it is helpful to obtain a second or third recording channel, which may reveal a clear underlying rhythm. If intrinsic QRS complexes are visible, calipers should be used to march out putative sinus QRS intervals. Wide-complex tachycardia caused by artifact may show a nonphysiologic rate or QRS duration. Other clues to artifact include presence of obvious motion artifact preceding the putative NSVT and absence of any pause preceding return of sinus rhythm.

Although ECG artifact might seem to be a trivial issue, it has been well documented to cause diagnostic confusion and serious errors in management.[6] Knight and colleagues[6] described a case series of 12 patients at an academic medical center who were misdiagnosed as having NSVT, whereas further review suggested artifact. Misdiagnoses were made by a cardiologist in 5 of the 12 cases and led to serious errors, including use of antiarrhythmic drugs, cardiac catheterization, and referrals for invasive electrophysiologic study and ICD placement. This important report underscores the importance of direct, first-hand review of the index tracing of putative NSVT by the consulting clinician before accepting the diagnosis in a consultation request.

Paced rhythm Paced rhythms may mimic the appearance of NSVT, particularly when a dual-chamber pacemaker or ICD in DDD mode is tracking sinus tachycardia, atrial tachycardia, or atrial flutter. Although a paced QRS complex is usually discerned easily on a 12-lead ECG, very small bipolar pacemaker artifact may not be apparent on a single-channel ambulatory ECG or

---

Box 1
Conditions that mimic NSVT

ECG artifact
- Loose electrode
- Motion/mechanical disturbance
- Tremor
- Electromagnetic interference

Paced rhythm
- Tracking sinus or atrial tachycardia in DDD mode
- Tracking artifact from fractured atrial lead
- Pacemaker-mediated tachycardia

Supraventricular arrhythmia with conduction aberrancy
- Typical bundle branch block aberrancy
  - Right bundle branch block
  - Left bundle branch block
  - Permanent versus rate related
- Preexcited tachycardia
  - Antidromic reciprocating tachycardia
  - Pathway-pathway reciprocating tachycardia
  - Supraventricular tachycardia with preexcitation
    - Irregular: atrial fibrillation
    - Regular: atrial tachycardia, atrioventricular (AV) node reentry tachycardia, atrial flutter

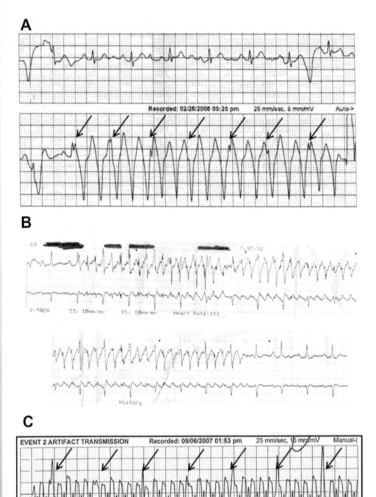

Fig. 3. ECG artifact mimicking NSVT. (*A*) Event monitor tracing from a 50-year-old woman with palpitations and lightheadedness that triggered an emergency call to the covering physician. The recording occurred while the patient was brushing her teeth. Sinus QRS complexes can be seen marching through the artifact (*arrows*). (*B*) Two-channel hospital telemetry recording triggering detection of supposed NSVT. The upper channel appears to show polymorphic VT, and the lower channel clearly shows sinus rhythm QRS complexes. (*C*) The tracing appears to show a rapid monomorphic VT with a cycle length of 160 milliseconds, which is nonphysiologic. On closer inspection, sinus QRS complexes can be marched out through the tracing (*arrows*).

telemetry tracing. In evaluating a patient who is a poor historian, it may occasionally be necessary to ascertain the presence of a pacemaker on physical examination or review of a chest radiograph. Erroneous tracking of artifact may also occur in the setting of an atrial lead fracture or electromagnetic interference when pacing in DDD mode (**Fig. 4**A).

In some circumstances, the pacemaker may create a reentrant loop, resulting in pacemaker-mediated tachycardia (PMT).[7] In this condition, a reentrant circuit forms when a ventricular depolarization is conducted in a retrograde fashion into the atria. The atrial lead senses the atrial depolarization, triggering a subsequent paced ventricular beat, which, in turn, is conducted in a retrograde fashion, establishing a reentrant circuit. PMT usually presents clinically as episodic ventricular pacing at the upper tracking rate of the pacemaker in DDD mode (usually 120–130 bpm). Because most pacemakers currently have features that automatically detect and terminate PMT, it typically presents as a nonsustained wide-complex arrhythmia that may mimic NSVT (**Fig. 4**B).

Supraventricular tachycardia with aberrancy Any form of SVT, including focal atrial tachycardia, orthodromic atrioventricular reciprocating tachycardia (AVRT), atrioventricular nodal reentrant tachycardia, atrial flutter, or atrial fibrillation, may conduct with aberrancy. This phenomenon usually results in a typical right bundle branch block (RBBB) or left bundle branch block (LBBB) QRS pattern. Bundle branch block in this setting may be caused by permanent or rate-related block in the corresponding bundle branch. Preexcited

A

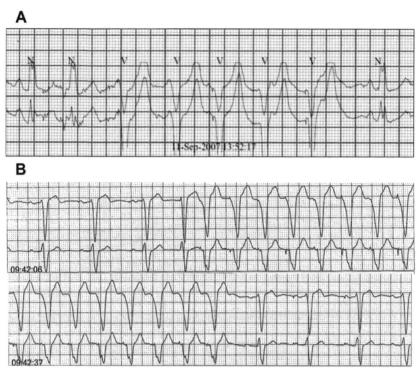

Fig. 4. Paced rhythm mimicking NSVT. (*A*) The figure is taken from an ambulatory ECG recording that led to consultation for NSVT. Further evaluation disclosed an atrial lead fracture and tracking of noise on the atrial channel in DDD mode. (*B*) Pacemaker-mediated tachycardia initially mistaken for NSVT. Pacemaker artifact is particularly difficult to discern in the upper channel.

tachycardia (antidromic AVRT, pathway-pathway reciprocating tachycardia, or SVT with preexcitation) is an increasingly uncommon form of wide-complex tachycardia that may mimic VT, because ventricular activation does not occur through the His-Purkinje system (**Fig. 5**).

Algorithms for distinguishing VT from SVT with aberrancy on 12-lead ECG have been described.[8,9] These algorithms are not validated for patients with congenital heart disease or for preexcited tachycardias. When only a single-channel rhythm strip is available, distinguishing the two may be more challenging. Identifying atrioventricular dissociation, if present, is particularly helpful in these cases, because it unequivocally establishes VT as the rhythm (**Fig. 6**).

Differentiate monomorphic from polymorphic ventricular tachycardia

Once alternative diagnoses have been ruled out and the diagnosis of NSVT has been made with sufficient certainty, the next step is to distinguish monomorphic VT from polymorphic VT (**Fig. 7**). Monomorphic VT is characterized by a regular rate with a very similar or identical appearance of each QRS complex. Occasionally, there are minor variations in QRS morphology caused by dissociated p-waves or baseline wander artifact. In contrast, polymorphic VT is characterized by an irregular rate, with varying morphology of each QRS complex.

Distinguishing between monomorphic and polymorphic VT is important for several reasons

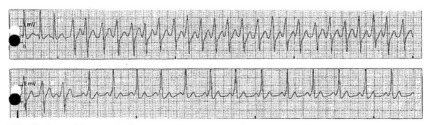

Fig. 5. Atrial fibrillation with ventricular preexcitation mimicking NSVT. A short PR interval and delta wave are apparent after sinus rhythm is restored in the lower portion of the tracing.

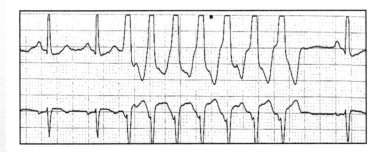

Fig. 6. NSVT with atrioventricular (AV) dissociation. Sinus p-waves are clearly seen marching through the wide-complex portion of the tracing, confirming the diagnosis of VT.

(Fig. 8).[10] The differential diagnosis for patients with monomorphic VT includes stable ischemic heart disease with remote myocardial infarction (MI) as well as other forms of cardiomyopathy, but may be idiopathic and associated with a structurally normal heart. In contrast, the differential diagnosis of polymorphic VT also includes acute coronary ischemia, long QT syndrome (LQTS), and other forms of inherited heart disease. Episodes of polymorphic VT, particularly if prolonged, are almost always associated with clinical instability and carry a malignant prognosis. In contrast, monomorphic VT may be associated with a stable perfusing blood pressure, even in prolonged episodes, and may have a benign prognosis in cases of idiopathic VT.

Further evaluation and therapy based on type of ventricular tachycardia and clinical circumstances

Once the distinction between monomorphic and polymorphic VT has been established, the clinician should pursue a focused and targeted evaluation based on the type of VT and clinical circumstances.

Evaluation of nonsustained polymorphic ventricular tachycardia

Proceeding first down the polymorphic VT pathway, the critical next step is to evaluate the sinus rhythm ECG to determine whether a prolonged QT interval with or without an abnormal T-wave morphology is present. Polymorphic VT occurring in the setting of a prolonged QT interval is defined as torsades de pointes and has a well-established differential diagnosis (Box 2).

Once an LQTS has been diagnosed, efforts should be made to ascertain whether the syndrome is inherited or acquired. Information on family history of arrhythmias, syncope, and premature sudden death; prior ECGs; review of medications; and determination of serum potassium and magnesium levels are particularly important in the evaluation.

Congenital LQTS typically presents at a younger age and may be associated with positive family history, usually in an autosomal dominant pattern (Fig. 9A). The QT interval usually remains prolonged on serial ECGs and arrhythmia may be precipitated by exercise, diving, or sudden alarm. Genetic evaluation may reveal mutations in 1 or more genes associated with cardiac repolarization in about 70% of established cases, and may be particularly useful for screening at-risk family members.[11,12] More recent data also suggest that genetic evaluation may be useful for establishing prognosis and determining therapy in the probands.[13,14]

Acquired LQTS is associated with older age, transient QT prolongation, absence of family history, and presence of 1 or more precipitants, particularly culprit medications, hypokalemia,

A

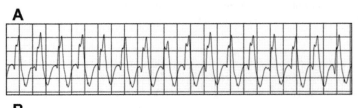

B

Fig. 7. Monomorphic and polymorphic VT. (A) Monomorphic VT is indicated by the regular rate and nearly identical QRS complexes. (B) Polymorphic VT is indicated by the varying cycle length and beat-to-beat variation in QRS morphology.

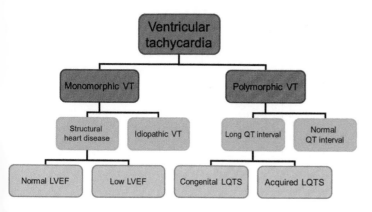

Fig. 8. Differentiation of monomorphic from polymorphic VT. The figure outlines a diagnostic pathway for evaluation of NSVT emphasizing the distinction between monomorphic and polymorphic VT. LQTS, long QT syndrome.

and hypomagnesemia (**Fig. 9**B). Medications most strongly associated with acquired LQTS include class IA (eg, quinidine, procainamide, disopyramide) and III (eg, sotalol, dofetilide, ibutilide) antiarrhythmic drugs.[15] Other culprit medications include certain fluoroquinolone and macrolide antibiotics and antipsychotic medications as well as methadone, particularly in high doses. AZCERT, Inc, maintains a list of medications associated with acquired LQTS at crediblemeds.org. Rare causes of acquired LQTS include pheochromocytoma, starvation, complete atrioventricular block, hypothyroidism, and central nervous system disease (**Fig. 9**C).[16]

Box 2
Causes of LQTS and NSVT/torsades de pointes

Congenital LQTS
- Mutations in genes mediating cardiac potassium currents I_{Kr} and I_{Ks}
  - LQT1, LQT2, LQT5, LQT6
- Mutations in genes mediating cardiac sodium current I_{Na}
  - LQT3
- Mutations in other genes (rare)
  - LQT4, LQT7 to LQT15

Acquired LQTS
- Medications
  - Antiarrhythmic medications (class IA and III)
  - Antibiotics (fluoroquinolones, erythromycins)
  - Antipsychotics
  - Methadone
  - Miscellaneous
- Electrolyte disturbances
  - Hypokalemia
  - Hypomagnesemia
- Complete AV block
- Acute neurologic disease
- Metabolic/endocrine disorders
  - Pheochromocytoma
  - Hypothyroidism
  - Anorexia/starvation

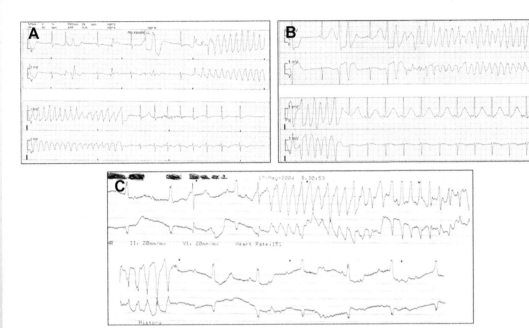

Fig. 9. Examples of LQTS and torsades de pointes. (*A*) A 40-year-old woman with congenital LQTS and family history of premature sudden death. (*B*) A 48-year-old woman treated with gatifloxacin, a fluoroquinolone antibiotic, for an ear infection in the setting of hypokalemia and hypomagnesemia. Echocardiogram showed a structurally normal heart. (*C*) Episode of torsades de pointes in a patient presenting with new complete AV block.

Distinguishing between NSVT caused by congenital and acquired LQTS is important for several reasons. Congenital LQTS confers a lifelong susceptibility to torsades de pointes and sudden death and may require lifelong therapy with β-blockers and an ICD in high-risk patients.[13] A diagnosis of congenital LQTS has important implications for genetic testing and for screening family members.[12] In contrast, acquired LQTS implies only transient risk and usually requires only removal/correction of the precipitating factors and observation, with use of intravenous magnesium and measures to increase heart rate in patients with NSVT/torsades de pointes. β-Blockers may be harmful in patients with acquired LQTS, because lower heart rates tend to predispose to torsades de pointes in this condition, and family members are not at significant risk and do not require screening. In both congenital and acquired LQTS, patients should avoid future exposure to medications associated with LQTS and torsades de pointes.[17]

For patients with polymorphic VT associated with a normal QT interval, the first consideration should be for evaluation for coronary ischemia (**Fig. 10, Box 3**). Because of the false-negative

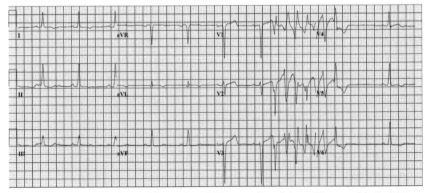

Fig. 10. Polymorphic VT in setting of unstable angina. ECG was taken from a 65-year-old woman recovering from pneumonia. Coronary angiography showed critical double-vessel CAD, which was treated with an intra-aortic balloon pump and urgent coronary artery bypass grafting.

Box 3
Causes of polymorphic NSVT with normal QT interval

Coronary ischemia
- ST elevation MI
- Non–ST elevation MI
- Unstable angina
- Coronary vasospasm
- Coronary dissection
- Congenital coronary anomaly

Cardiomyopathy
- Ischemic/postinfarction cardiomyopathy
- Nonischemic cardiomyopathy
  - Idiopathic dilated cardiomyopathy
  - Cardiomyopathy caused by valvular heart disease
  - Infiltrative cardiomyopathy
    - Cardiac sarcoidosis
    - Cardiac amyloidosis
  - Myocarditis

Inherited/genetic electrical heart disease
- Congenital LQTS with normal QT
- Brugada syndrome
- Catecholaminergic polymorphic VT
- Short QT syndrome
- Sudden cardiac death/ventricular fibrillation (VF) with early repolarization
- Other idiopathic VF

---

rate, functional stress testing is often insufficient to exclude a life-threatening coronary lesion in this clinical situation. Proceeding directly to cardiac catheterization is reasonable in patients with known CAD or substantial risk factors. For lower-risk patients, or in young patients in whom congenital coronary anomaly is an important consideration, coronary computed tomography (CT) angiography may be appropriate.

Evaluation of left ventricular (LV) function should be undertaken in all patients with nonsustained polymorphic VT, usually with echocardiography, which is an excellent modality for excluding other important cardiac disorders such as hypertrophic cardiomyopathy and valvular heart disease. If structural heart disease is not fully excluded with ECG and echocardiography, then further evaluation with cardiac MRI may be considered. Cardiac MRI is a particularly good modality for evaluation of right ventricular morphology and function and to evaluate for atypical forms of hypertrophic cardiomyopathy with minimal or absent septal and basal LV wall thickening.[18,19] Use of gadolinium contrast allows for assessment of delayed myocardial enhancement, which typically indicates areas of cardiac scarring and/or inflammation and may be seen in a wide variety of cardiomyopathies, including myocarditis and cardiac sarcoidosis.[20,21] Identification of significant structural heart disease with any of the tests discussed earlier should lead to further evaluation and therapy, which is beyond the scope of this article.

If no structural heart disease is identified after thorough evaluation, patients with nonsustained polymorphic VT and normal QT interval may have a form of inherited electrical heart disease.[22] Patients with congenital LQTS occasionally present with a normal QT interval. Brugada syndrome is diagnosed when characteristic coved ST segment elevation is present in the right precordial leads.[23] When the diagnosis of Brugada syndrome is suspected but a type I patterns is not present on the baseline ECG, a challenge with intravenous sodium channel blocker, such as procainamide, flecainide, or ajmaline, may be performed. Genetic testing may not be helpful in equivocal cases, because definite mutations are seen in only a minority of cases of confirmed Brugada syndrome, and the diagnostic confusion created by identification of genetic variants of uncertain significance is being increasing recognized.[24] Catecholaminergic polymorphic VT (CPVT) is a rare syndrome that usually presents in children and young adults with normal resting ECG and echocardiography.[25] Ventricular arrhythmia is typically elicited with exercise testing. Bidirectional VT, a nearly pathognomonic feature of CPVT, may also be seen. As with Brugada syndrome, genetic testing in the absence of a clear clinical diagnosis or the context of family cascade screening is usually not clinically helpful.

In recent years, a potential risk of ventricular arrhythmia and sudden death associated with early repolarization has been recognized, particularly in cases of greater than 2 mm ST elevation in the inferior limb leads. Although previously thought to represent a common and benign ECG variant, early repolarization has been found to be more prevalent in young survivors of idiopathic ventricular fibrillation (VF) and to be associated with greater risk of recurrence of VF.[26] Early repolarization was also associated with a higher risk of cardiac death in a large longitudinal population study, although the absolute risk is low.[27] The

prognosis and best treatment of patients with NSVT and early repolarization is currently unknown.[28] Additional forms of idiopathic VF will likely be defined in future years.

Evaluation of nonsustained monomorphic ventricular tachycardia

An overview of the diagnostic considerations for patients with nonsustained monomorphic VT is given in **Fig. 11**. As with patients who have nonsustained polymorphic VT associated with a normal QT interval, assessment for evidence of structural heart disease is essential, starting with careful review of the 12-lead ECG and two-dimensional echocardiography.[29] In contrast with polymorphic VT, monomorphic VT is rarely a presenting feature of acute or critical coronary ischemia and is much more commonly seen late after MI in patients with otherwise stable CAD. The process by which MI leads to myocardial scarring and forms the substrate for monomorphic VT has been well described, as has the associated risk for sudden death.[30]

Myocardial substrates for monomorphic VT associated with structural heart disease may be divided into those with normal LV ejection fraction (LVEF) ($\geq$50%) and those with reduced LVEF (<50%) (**Box 4**). Those patients with reduced LVEF include patients with ischemic cardiomyopathy caused by prior MI and patients with nonischemic cardiomyopathy. The latter group

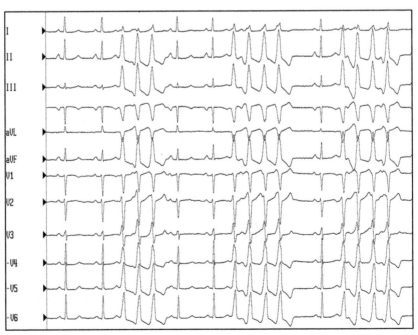

Fig. 11. NSVT originating in the right ventricular outflow tract (RVOT). Narrow QRS NSVT with a typical LBBB/inferior axis morphology is seen.

Box 4
Causes of monomorphic NSVT

Reduced LVEF

- Ischemic/postinfarction cardiomyopathy
- Nonischemic cardiomyopathy
  - Idiopathic dilated cardiomyopathy
  - Cardiomyopathy caused by valvular heart disease
  - Infiltrative cardiomyopathy
    - Cardiac sarcoidosis
    - Cardiac amyloidosis
  - Myocarditis

Normal LVEF

- Structural heart disease present
  - Hypertrophic cardiomyopathy
  - Arrhythmogenic right ventricular dysplasia/cardiomyopathy
  - Infiltrative cardiomyopathy
  - Mitral valve prolapse
  - Hypertensive heart disease
- Structural heart disease absent (idiopathic VT)

includes patients with idiopathic dilated cardiomyopathy, myocarditis, and cardiac sarcoidosis. Discussion of the evaluation and treatment of these clinical scenarios is beyond the scope of this article, but may include cardiac MRI, PET-CT scanning, coronary angiography, endomyocardial biopsy, and electrophysiologic study. A primary goal of treatment is risk stratification for sudden arrhythmic death and treatment of high-risk patients with a primary prevention ICD.

Patients with NSVT and structural heart disease with normal LVEF may include patients with hypertrophic cardiomyopathy, arrhythmogenic right ventricular dysplasia (ARVD)/cardiomyopathy, and infiltrative cardiomyopathies such as cardiac sarcoidosis. In each of these cases, the presence of NSVT increases the risk of sudden death and should be considered in risk stratification.[31–33] NSVT may occur in patients with mitral valve prolapse, but its association with risk of sudden death has not been well established in this context.[34] Although the presence of NSVT in patients with chronic arterial hypertension has raised concern, studies have not shown a consistent pattern of increased risk in patients without CAD.[35–37] When associated LV hypertrophy (LVH) is present, effective antihypertensive therapy, which may include a β-blocker, is especially important to

reduce cardiovascular risk.[38] Monomorphic VT is rarely a presenting feature of inherited electrical heart disease.

Idiopathic Ventricular Tachycardia

When monomorphic VT occurs in the absence of structural heart disease, idiopathic VT is diagnosed. This condition usually presents in young adults, but may be seen in children and elderly patients as well. Symptoms of idiopathic VT may include palpitations, lightheadedness, chest discomfort, and syncope. The prognosis is favorable, and reliable reports of sudden death are extremely rare.

Outflow tract ventricular tachycardia

Several variants of idiopathic VT have been described, the most common of which is outflow tract VT (**Box 5**). These arrhythmias have a focal mechanism, most commonly originating in the right ventricular outflow tract (RVOT), and have an LBBB/inferior axis morphology with a narrow QRS (**Fig. 11**). VTs originating in the LV outflow tract and aortic root (right/left coronary cusps, aortomitral continuity) have increasingly been reported, and these may have an LBBB pattern with early precordial transition or RBBB morphology (**Fig. 12**). More detailed algorithms for determining site of origin of outflow tract VTs based on surface ECG morphology have been described.[39,40]

Box 5
Idiopathic VT: most common sites of origin

Outflow tract VT

- Right ventricular outflow tract
- LV outflow tract
- Aortic root/coronary cusp
  - Right coronary cusp
  - Left coronary cusp
- Aortomitral continuity
- Great cardiac vein

Fascicular VT

- Left anterior fascicular VT
- Left posterior fascicular VT

Papillary muscle

- LV papillary muscles
  - With mitral valve prolapse
  - Without mitral valve prolapse
- Right ventricular papillary muscles

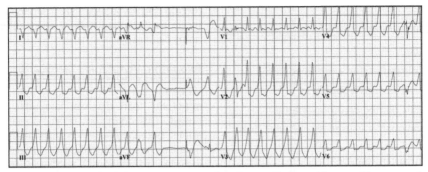

Fig. 12. NSVT originating from the left coronary cusp. Taken from a 62-year-old man with recurrent palpitations. QRS morphology is RBBB/inferior axis with positive precordial concordance.

Outflow tract VTs have a variety of presentations. Patients may have sustained VT, which can be exercised induced. Other patients have a pattern of nearly incessant short bursts of NSVT (**Fig. 13**). Still other patients have a predominant pattern of frequent premature ventricular contractions (PVCs). The last 2 scenarios may result in LV dysfunction and heart failure, particularly when the total burden of ventricular ectopy exceeds about 25% of all QRS complexes on 24-hour ambulatory ECG monitoring.[41] LV dysfunction may result from chronic dyssynchronous LV contraction, similar to the pathophysiology of chronic LBBB, but the exact pathogenesis has not been determined. Catheter ablation of outflow tract ventricular arrhythmias has been shown to improve LV function in these patients.[38]

When patients with apparently normal hearts present with NSVT that has an LBBB morphology, ARVD and cardiac sarcoidosis should be considered.[42] For patients with a single morphology of typical LBBB/inferior axis VT without malignant symptoms or family history and with a normal baseline ECG and echocardiogram, additional evaluation has a low yield.[43,44] For patients with testing abnormalities, more than 1 morphology of VT, or VT with morphology atypical for RVOT origin, further evaluation with cardiac MRI, PET-CT, and/or signal-averaged ECG should be considered. ARVD should be diagnosed using Task Force criteria, rather than based on a single test or clinical scenario.[32] Cardiac sarcoidosis may mimic ARVD in some patients with right ventricular predominance and arrhythmia of right ventricular origin.[45]

Patients with idiopathic outflow tract VT may be treated with a variety of medications, including β-blockers, diltiazem, verapamil, and class IC or III antiarrhythmic agents, depending on the clinical circumstances.[38] The effective medication with the lowest side effect profile for a given patient should be considered. For patients with frequent, repetitive NSVT causing symptoms of LV dysfunction or patients with symptomatic inducible sustained VT, catheter ablation is an effective alternative (**Fig. 14**).[46]

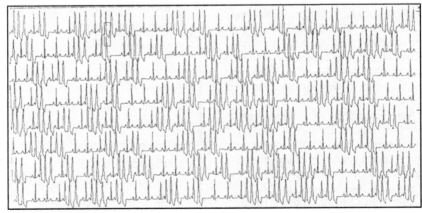

Fig. 13. Repetitive monomorphic VT. Incessant NSVT originating in the outflow tract region. Ventricular complexes make up more than 50% of total QRS complexes on the tracing.

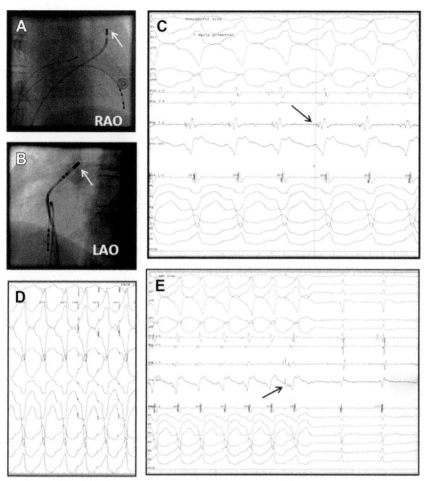

Fig. 14. Catheter ablation of RVOT VT. (*A, B*) The ablation catheter is positioned just below the pulmonic valve on the anterior septal RVOT (*arrows*). (*C*) Activation mapping shows presystolic electrogram on the distal ablation catheter with fractionated early component (*arrow*). (*D*) Pacing at the successful site shows that the paced QRS morphology (last 3 beats) is identical to the VT morphology (*E*) Radiofrequency energy application (*arrow*) results in termination of sustained VT in a single beat. RAO, right anterior oblique view; LAO, left anterior oblique view.

Malignant form of outflow tract ventricular tachycardia

Several reports have raised concerns of a malignant form of outflow tract arrhythmia, usually short-coupled PVCs triggering idiopathic VF.[47,48] One report, by Noda and colleagues,[49] examined 101 patients without structural heart disease undergoing catheter ablation for idiopathic RVOT arrhythmias and found 16 patients who had spontaneous episodes of VF (n = 5) or unexplained syncope (n = 11).[49] Holter monitoring showed RVOT-morphology PVCs initiating polymorphic VT with rapid cycle length (mean 245 ± 28 milliseconds) in each patient. Seven of these 16 patients also had monomorphic NSVT with a fairly rapid mean cycle length of 273 ± 23 milliseconds.[50] By comparison, patients with benign RVOT VT (n = 85) had slower mean cycle

length of 328 ± 65 milliseconds and a monomorphic form of VT. No patient was reported to have only monomorphic VT leading to VF.

Overall, the medical literature suggests that patients with only monomorphic NSVT with RVOT morphology have a very low risk of fatal outcome if structural and inherited heart disease is definitively excluded. In some patients with atypical clinical or ECG features, serial follow-up imaging and/or ECG monitoring may be warranted to exclude development of structural heart disease or additional forms of VT.

Fascicular ventricular tachycardia

The second most common form of idiopathic VT is fascicular VT, a form of ventricular arrhythmia that uses the His-Purkinje system and usually takes an RBBB/superior axis morphology[51] (**Fig. 15**). Less

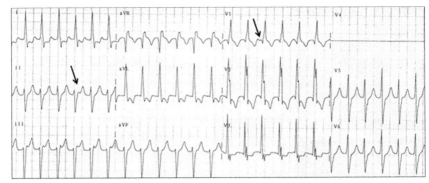

Fig. 15. Idiopathic left anterior fascicular VT. QRS duration is short and morphology is RBBB/superior axis. This arrhythmia is often mistaken for SVT with aberrancy. In this case, AV dissociation is clearly seen on the tracing (*arrows*).

commonly, an RBBB/inferior axis QRS morphology is seen. Evidence suggests that this arrhythmia involves microreentry using components of the left bundle branch, but the exact mechanism has not been definitively established. The arrhythmia is characteristically sensitive to intravenous verapamil acutely; oral verapamil seems moderately effective for chronic suppression. For patients with RBBB/superior axis fascicular VT, endocardial ablation in the left ventricle in the region of the left posterior fascicle is usually successful for long-term suppression.[46,52]

Papillary muscle ventricular tachycardia

More recently, an additional form of idiopathic VT arising from ventricular papillary muscles has been described (**Fig. 16**). Doppalapudi and colleagues[53] reported 7 patients in a series of 290 patients referred for idiopathic VT (2.4%) with VT or frequent PVCs arising from the base of the

posterior LV papillary muscle. All patients had normal LVEF, although 2 had CAD. ECGs showed RBBB/superior axis VT in all patients. All appeared to have a focal mechanism and most were associated with exercise and induced with catecholamines in the electrophysiology (EP) laboratory. None appeared to originate from the His-Purkinje system and all required irrigated ablation for successful elimination. Subsequent reports have documented idiopathic VT originating from the anterior LV papillary muscle and from right ventricular papillary muscles.[54,55]

Nonsustained ventricular tachycardia in patients with hypertension

Epidemiologic studies have shown that the presence of arterial hypertension increases risk of all-cause mortality and sudden death, particularly when associated with LVH. Other studies have shown that hypertensive heart disease,

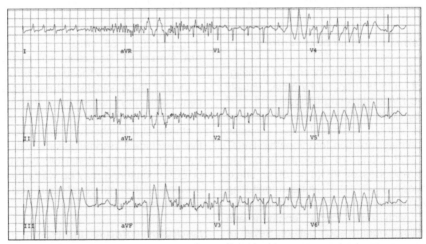

Fig. 16. Papillary muscle NSVT. A 21-year-old woman with mild mitral valve prolapse whose ECG during exercise shows runs of NSVT with an RBBB/superior axis morphology with a late precordial transition. The QRS duration is fairly wide and there is some slight beat-to-beat variation. EP study confirms focal VT from the posterior papillary muscle induced with isoproterenol.

particularly LVH, is associated with ventricular arrhythmias.[56,57] McLenachan and colleagues[58] studied 100 patients with hypertension at an outpatient clinic in the United Kingdom, half of whom had LVH by ECG criteria, and 50 normotensive control subjects. They found NSVT in 28% of patients with hypertension and LVH, 8% of patients with hypertension and no LVH, and 2% of control subjects. In addition, hypertensive patients with NSVT had substantially greater LV mass by echocardiography than those without NSVT. This study established a clear link between hypertensive LVH and development of NSVT. Other smaller studies suggested that regression of LVH with antihypertensive treatment is associated with a reduction in ventricular arrhythmias.[59]

Data on the prognostic significance of NSVT in patients with hypertension are mixed. Galinier and colleagues[37] examined 214 hypertensive patients with mean age of 59 years, one-third of whom had LVH by echocardiography. Thirty-three (16.2%) of the patients had NSVT. NSVT was a significant predictor of risk of total mortality (relative risk [RR] = 2.6) and cardiac death (RR = 3.5). Other studies have failed to show increased risk posed by presence of NSVT in hypertensive patients.[60] Seth and colleagues[61] reviewed records of 1125 enrollees in a pacemaker clinic (nearly 80% of patients with hypertension) and found no increased risk of long-term mortality in the 20% of patients who had NSVT.

Overall, it has been established that hypertension, especially when associated with LVH, is associated with increased risk of NSVT and mortality, but it is not clear that ventricular arrhythmia increases mortality risk independently. Therefore, diagnosis and management of NSVT in this population should proceed similarly to the algorithm suggested earlier. Distinguishing patients with hypertensive LVH from those with hypertrophic cardiomyopathy sometimes poses a particular challenge. Attention to good control of hypertension is important. When symptomatic NSVT requires treatment, a β-blocker is a reasonable first choice. Because of risk of proarrhythmia, most antiarrhythmic drugs should be used with caution in patients with hypertension and moderate or severe LVH.

Nonsustained ventricular tachycardia in athletes

Sudden cardiac death in young athletes, although rare, is a traumatic event that can affect entire communities. It has led to heightened health screening and surveillance, particularly for college, professional, and elite amateur athletes, which may lead to identification of NSVT. The Seattle Criteria for classification of ECG findings in athletes considers NSVT to be an abnormality requiring further evaluation.[62] NSVT in this setting therefore warrants careful evaluation according to the algorithm described earlier in the article, with particular attention to the exclusion of structural and inherited heart disease, such as hypertrophic cardiomyopathy and ARVD. Athletes should also be asked about the use of performance-enhancing and other illicit drugs.

High-intensity physical exercise may lead to morphologic and electrical changes that have been termed athlete's heart.[63] A few investigators have raised concern that endurance training may produce acute and chronic right ventricular (RV) dysfunction that may promote ventricular arrhythmias in otherwise normal athletic hearts.[64] Heidbuchel[65] reported on 46 high-level endurance athletes (80% cyclists) with ventricular arrhythmias (24 [52%] with NSVT) followed for a mean of 4.7 years. Eighty percent of ventricular arrhythmias had an LBBB morphology, suggesting RV origin. Eighteen athletes (39%) had major arrhythmic events, including 9 (20%) with sudden death. Athletes with arrhythmic events were younger and more likely to have inducible VT or VF at EP study. Presence of NSVT was not predictive of events. Although this study is concerning, it may be explained by referral bias and failure to identify structural or inherited heart disease. It has not been corroborated by other reports.

In the absence of more data suggesting arrhythmic risk posed by athletes' hearts, NSVT in athletes should require the same diagnostic and therapeutic approach described earlier. Given that idiopathic VT may be induced by exercise and athletic performance may be affected by antiarrhythmic medications, a curative ablative approach may be preferred by athletic patients with symptomatic arrhythmia.

Exercise-induced nonsustained ventricular tachycardia

NSVT that is seen during exercise, whether recorded on ambulatory ECG monitor or during clinical exercise testing, should be approached similarly according to the algorithm described earlier. For patients with polymorphic ventricular arrhythmia, first consideration should be given to evaluation for coronary ischemia and other forms of structural heart disease. CPVT and other forms of inherited arrhythmia syndromes, although rare, may also present in this setting. For patients with monomorphic VT with exercise, examination of 12-lead QRS morphology can be helpful in localizing the site of origin and narrowing the differential diagnosis. As with patients with polymorphic VT, a careful search for evidence of structural heart disease should be undertaken before a diagnosis of idiopathic VT is made, particularly for patients in whom the 12-lead ECG features are atypical.

Several studies have addressed the prognostic significance of exercise-induced nonsustained ventricular arrhythmia, including NSVT. Jouven and colleagues[66] examined the results of exercise tests in 6101 asymptomatic middle-aged French civil servants with a mean follow-up of 23 years. Over a mean follow-up of 23 years, complex exercise-induced ventricular arrhythmia (defined as 2 or more consecutive beats or >10% of total beats) predicted total and cardiovascular mortality. Frolkis and colleagues[67] reviewed exercise tests for 29,244 patients undergoing exercise testing for clinical indications and found over a mean follow-up of 5.3 years that exercise-induced ventricular arrhythmia (frequent ventricular premature depolarizations, bigeminy, couplets, or NSVT) was associated with increased mortality (hazard ratio, 1.8) on univariate analysis. However, after propensity matching for confounding variables, only complex ventricular arrhythmia during recovery (and not during exercise) predicted increased mortality. Eckart and colleagues[68] reviewed 585 patients with exercise-induced ventricular arrhythmia (defined as couplets, triplets, or multifocal ectopy) during clinically indicated exercise testing and compared outcomes with 2340 matched controls over a mean follow-up of 2 years. Exercise-induced ventricular arrhythmia with RBBB morphology or multiple morphologies predicted higher mortality, whereas ventricular arrhythmia with left bundle branch morphology did not.

Yang and colleagues[69] found that exercise-induced NSVT developed in 50 (1.5%) of 3.351 patients (mean age, 62 years) undergoing clinically indicated exercise testing. NSVT episodes were usually brief, with 60% having only 3 beats. Over a mean follow-up of 26 months, there was no difference in outcomes between those patients with and without NSVT.

Another study investigated a population of healthy older volunteers participating in the Baltimore Longitudinal Study of Aging.[70] A total of 2099 subjects (mean age, 52 years; 52% male) underwent treadmill exercise testing and 79 (3.7%) developed NSVT of 3 or more beats (84% ≤5 beats; median rate, 175 bpm). Subjects with exercise-induced NSVT were older and more likely to be male. There was a marked increase in prevalence of exercise-induced NSVT with age, with prevalence more than 10% in men more than 70 years of age. Over a mean follow-up of 13.5 years, there was no difference in total

mortality after multivariable adjustment. The study concluded that brief asymptomatic runs of NSVT in the absence of clinical heart disease are not rare in older adults and generally do not carry an adverse prognosis.

SUMMARY

NSVT is a common cause for cardiology and EP consultation and is present in at least 0.5% to 1% of healthy adults with at least 1 ambulatory ECG recording. Establishing the presence or absence of structural or inherited heart disease is a critical step in each patient's evaluation. This article describes a systematic approach to the evaluation of NSVT. Conditions that may mimic the appearance of NSVT should be excluded, and monomorphic VT and polymorphic VT should be distinguished from one another. Patients should be carefully evaluated for acute ischemia, structural heart disease, and inherited electrical heart disease before concluding that they have normal hearts. When nonsustained monomorphic VT occurs in a patient with a normal heart, a form of idiopathic VT is usually diagnosed. Treatment is targeted toward symptoms, and may consist of observation, medical therapy, or catheter ablation, depending on the frequency and severity of symptoms and the clinical situation.

REFERENCES

1. Bikkina M, Larson MG, Levy D. Prognostic implications of asymptomatic ventricular arrhythmias: the Framingham Heart Study. Ann Intern Med 1992; 117:990–6.

2. Hingorani P, Karnad DR, Rohekar P, et al. Arrhythmias seen in baseline 24-hour Holter ECG recordings in healthy normal volunteers during phase I clinical trials. J Clin Pharmacol 2015. http://dx.doi.org/10.1002/jcph.679.

3. Bigger JT, Fleiss JL, Rolnitzky LM. Prevalence, characteristics and significance of ventricular tachycardia detected by 24-hour continuous electrocardiographic recordings in the late hospital phase of acute myocardial infarction. Am J Cardiol 1986;58:1151–60.

4. De Sousa MR, Morillo CA, Rabelo FT, et al. Nonsustained ventricular tachycardia as a predictor of sudden cardiac death in patients with left ventricular dysfunction: a meta-analysis. Eur J Heart Fail 2008; 10:1007–14.

5. Katritsis DG, Zareba W, Camm AJ. Nonsustained ventricular tachycardia. J Am Coll Cardiol 2012;60: 1993–2004.

6. Knight BP, Pelosi F, Michaud GF, et al. Clinical consequences of electrocardiographic artifact mimicking

ventricular tachycardia. N Engl J Med 1999;341:
1270–4.

7. Monteil B, Ploux S, Eschalier R, et al. Pacemaker-mediated tachycardia: manufacturer specifics and spectrum of cases. Pacing Clin Electrophysiol 2015;38:1489–98.

8. Brugada P, Brugada J, Mont L, et al. A new approach to the differential diagnosis of a regular tachycardia with a wide QRS complex. Circulation 1991;83:1649–59.

9. Vereckei A, Duray G, Szenasi G, et al. Application of a new algorithm in the differential diagnosis of wide QRS complex tachycardia. Eur Heart J 2007;28: 589–600.

10. Prystowsky EN, Padanilam BJ, Joshi S, et al. Ventricular arrhythmias in the absence of structural heart disease. J Am Coll Cardiol 2012;59: 1733–44.

11. Nakano Y, Shimizu W. Genetics of long-QT syndrome. J Hum Genet 2015. http://dx.doi.org/10. 1038/jhg.2015.74.

12. Ackerman MJ, Priori SG, Willems S, et al. HRS/EHRA expert consensus statement on the state of genetic testing for the channelopathies and cardiomyopathies. Heart Rhythm 2011;8:1308–39.

13. Priori SG, Wilde AA, Horie M, et al. HRS/EHRA/APHRS expert consensus statement on the diagnosis and management of patients with inherited primary arrhythmia syndromes. Heart Rhythm 2013;10:1932–63.

14. Giudicessi JR, Ackerman MJ. Genotype- and phenotype-guided management of congenital long QT syndrome. Curr Probl Cardiol 2013;38: 417–55.

15. Yap YG, Camm AJ. Drug-induced QT prolongation and torsades de pointes. Heart 2003;89:1363–72.

16. Choudhuri I, Pinninti M, Marwali MR, et al. Polymorphic ventricular tachycardia–part I: structural heart disease and acquired causes. Curr Probl Cardiol 2013;38:463–96.

17. Available at: https://crediblemeds.org/. Accessed January 15, 2016.

18. Rastegar N, Burt JR, Corona-Villalobos CP, et al. Cardiac MR findings and potential diagnostic pitfalls in patients evaluated for arrhythmogenic right ventricular cardiomyopathy. Radiographics 2014;34: 1553–70.

19. Bogaert J, Olivotto I. MR imaging in hypertrophic cardiomyopathy: from magnet to bedside. Radiology 2014;273:329–48.

20. Saeed M, Van TA, Krug R, et al. Cardiac MR imaging: current status and future directions. Cardiovasc Diagn Ther 2015;5:290–310.

21. Aggarwal NR, Snipelisky D, Young PM, et al. Advances in imaging for diagnosis and management of cardiac sarcoidosis. Eur Heart J Cardiovasc Imaging 2015;16:949–58.

22. Choudhuri I, Pinninti M, Marwali MR, et al. Polymorphic ventricular tachycardia–Part II: the channelopathies. Curr Probl Cardiol 2013;38:503–48.

23. Brugada P, Brugada J, Roy D. Brugada syndrome 1992-2012: 20 years of scientific excitement, and more. Eur Heart J 2013;34:3610–5.

24. Ackerman MJ. Genetic purgatory and the cardiac channelopathies: exposing the variants of uncertain/unknown significance issue. Heart Rhythm 2015;12:2325–31.

25. van der Werf C, Wilde AA. Catecholaminergic polymorphic ventricular tachycardia: from bench to bedside. Heart 2013;99:497–504.

26. Haissaguerre M, Derval N, Sacher F, et al. Sudden cardiac arrest associated with early repolarization. N Engl J Med 2008;358:2016–23.

27. Tikannen JT, Anttonen O, Junttila MJ, et al. Long-term outcome associated with early repolarization on electrocardiography. N Engl J Med 2009;361:2529.

28. Obeyesekere MN, Klein GJ, Nattel S, et al. A clinical approach to early repolarization. Circulation 2013; 127:1620.

29. Marine JE. ECG features that suggest a potentially life-threatening arrhythmia as the cause for syncope. J Electrocardiol 2013;46:561–8.

30. Raymond JM, Sacher F, Winslow R, et al. Catheter ablation for scar-related ventricular tachycardias. Curr Probl Cardiol 2009;34:225–70.

31. Monserrat L, Elliott PM, Gimeno JR, et al. Non-sustained ventricular tachycardia in hypertrophic cardiomyopathy: an independent marker of sudden death risk in young patients. J Am Coll Cardiol 2003;42:873–9.

32. Marcus FI, McKenna WJ, Sherrill D, et al. Diagnosis of arrhythmogenic right ventricular cardiomyopathy/dysplasia: proposed modification of the Task Force criteria. Circulation 2010;121:1533–41.

33. Birnie DH, Sauer WH, Bogun F, et al. HRS expert consensus statement on the diagnosis and management of arrhythmias associated with cardiac sarcoidosis. Heart Rhythm 2014;11:1305–23.

34. Hayek E, Gring CN, Griffin BP. Mitral valve prolapse. Lancet 2005;365:507–18.

35. Pringle SD, Dunn FG, Macfarlane PW, et al. Significance of ventricular arrhythmias in systemic hypertension with left ventricular hypertrophy. Am J Cardiol 1992;69:913–7.

36. Bikkina M, Larson MG, Levy D. Asymptomatic ventricular arrhythmias and mortality risk in subjects with left ventricular hypertrophy. J Am Coll Cardiol 1993;22:1111–6.

37. Galinier M, Balanescu S, Fourcade J, et al. Prognostic value of ventricular arrhythmias in systemic hypertension. J Hypertens 1997;14:1779–83.

38. Pedersen CT, Kay GN, Kalman J, et al. EHRA/HRS/APHRS expert consensus on ventricular arrhythmias. Heart Rhythm 2014;11:e166–96.

39. Dixit S, Gerstenfeld EP, Callans DJ, et al. Electrocardiographic patterns of superior right ventricular outflow tract tachycardias: distinguishing septal and free-wall sites of origin. J Cardiovasc Electrophysiol 2003;14:1–7.

40. Betensky BP, Park RE, Marchlinski FE, et al. The V(2) transition ratio: a new electrocardiographic criterion for distinguishing left from right ventricular outflow tract tachycardia origin. J Am Coll Cardiol 2011;57:2255–62.

41. Bogun F, Crawford T, Reich S, et al. Radiofrequency ablation of frequent, idiopathic premature ventricular complexes: comparison with a control group without intervention. Heart Rhythm 2007;4:863–7.

42. Hoffmayer KS, Bhave PD, Marcus GM, et al. An electrocardiographic scoring system for distinguishing right ventricular outflow tract arrhythmias in patients with arrhythmogenic right ventricular cardiomyopathy from idiopathic ventricular tachycardia. Heart Rhythm 2013;10:477–82.

43. Nasir K, Bomma C, Tandri H, et al. Electrocardiographic features of arrhythmogenic right ventricular dysplasia/cardiomyopathy according to disease severity: a need to broaden diagnostic criteria. Circulation 2004;110:1527–34.

44. Yoerger DM, Marcus F, Sherrill D, et al. Echocardiographic findings in patients meeting Task Force criteria for arrhythmogenic right ventricular dysplasia: new insights from the multidisciplinary study of right ventricular dysplasia. J Am Coll Cardiol 2005;45:860–5.

45. Philips B, Madhavan S, James CA, et al. Arrhythmogenic right ventricular dysplasia/cardiomyopathy and cardiac sarcoidosis: distinguishing features when the diagnosis is unclear. Circ Arrhythm Electrophysiol 2014;7:230–6.

46. Aliot EM, Stevenson WG, Almendral-Garrote JM, et al. EHRA/HRS expert consensus on catheter ablation of ventricular arrhythmias. Heart Rhythm 2009;6:886–933.

47. Haissaguerre M, Shoda M, Jais P, et al. Mapping and ablation of idiopathic ventricular fibrillation. Circulation 2002;106:962–7.

48. Viskin S, Rosso R, Rogowski O, et al. The "short-coupled" variant of right ventricular outflow ventricular tachycardia: a not-so-benign form of benign ventricular tachycardia? J Cardiovasc Electrophysiol 2005;16:912–6.

49. Noda T, Shimizu W, Taguchi A, et al. Malignant entity of idiopathic ventricular fibrillation and polymorphic ventricular tachycardia initiated by premature extrasystoles originating from the right ventricular outflow tract. J Am Coll Cardiol 2005;46:1288–94.

50. Shimizu W. Arrhythmias originating from the right ventricular outflow tract: how to distinguish "malignant" from "benign"? Heart Rhythm 2009;6:1507–11.

51. Nogami A. Purkinje-related arrhythmias part I: monomorphic ventricular tachycardias. Pacing Clin Electrophysiol 2011;34:624–50.

52. Wissner E, Menon SY, Metzner A, et al. Long-term outcome after catheter ablation for left posterior fascicular ventricular tachycardia without development of left posterior fascicular block. J Cardiovasc Electrophysiol 2012;23:1179–84.

53. Doppalapudi H, Yamada T, McElderry HT, et al. Ventricular tachycardia originating from the posterior papillary muscle in the left ventricle: a distinct clinical syndrome. Circ Arrhythm Electrophysiol 2008;1:23–9.

54. Yamada T, McElderry HT, Okada T, et al. Idiopathic focal ventricular arrhythmias originating from the anterior papillary muscle in the left ventricle. J Cardiovasc Electrophysiol 2009;20:866–72.

55. Crawford T, Mueller G, Good E, et al. Ventricular arrhythmias originating from papillary muscles in the right ventricle. Heart Rhythm 2010;7:725–30.

56. Hennersdorf MG, Strauer BE. Arterial hypertension and cardiac arrhythmias. J Hypertens 2001;19:167–77.

57. Almendral J, Villacastin JP, Arenal A, et al. Evidence favoring the hypothesis that ventricular arrhythmias have prognostic significance in left ventricular hypertrophy secondary to systemic hypertension. Am J Cardiol 1995;76:60D–3D.

58. McLenachan JM, Henderson E, Morris KI, et al. Ventricular arrhythmias in patients with hypertensive left ventricular hypertrophy. N Engl J Med 1987;317:787–92.

59. Messerli FH, Nunez BD, Nunez MM, et al. Hypertension and sudden death: disparate effects of calcium entry blocker and diuretic therapy on cardiac dysrhythmias. Arch Intern Med 1989;149:1263–7.

60. Dunn FG, Pringle SD. Sudden cardiac death, ventricular arrhythmias, and hypertensive left ventricular hypertrophy. J Hypertens 1993;11:1003–10.

61. Seth N, Kaplan R, Bustamante E, et al. Clinical significance of nonsustained ventricular tachycardia on routine monitoring of pacemaker patients. Pacing Clin Electrophysiol 2015;38:980–8.

62. Drezner JA, Ackerman MJ, Anderson J, et al. Electrocardiographic interpretation in athletes: the 'Seattle' criteria. Br J Sports Med 2013;47:122–4.

63. Sharma S, Merghani A, Mont L. Exercise and the heart: the good, the bad, and the ugly. Eur Heart J 2015;36:1445–53.

64. La Gerche A, Burns AT, Mooney DJ, et al. Exercise-induced right ventricular dysfunction and structural remodelling in endurance athletes. Eur Heart J 2012;33:998–1006.

65. Heidbuchel H. High prevalence of right ventricular involvement in endurance athletes with ventricular arrhythmias role of an electrophysiologic study in risk stratification. Eur Heart J 2003;24:1473–80.

66. Jouven X, Zureik M, Desnos M, et al. Long-term outcome in asymptomatic men with exercise-induced premature ventricular depolarizations. N Engl J Med 2000;343:826–33.

67. Frolkis JP, Pothier CE, Blackstone EH, et al. Frequent ventricular ectopy after exercise as a predictor of death. N Engl J Med 2003;348:781–90.

68. Eckart RE, Field ME, Hruczkowski TW, et al. Association of electrocardiographic morphology of exercise ventricular arrhythmia with mortality. Ann Intern Med 2008;149:451–60.

69. Yang JC, Wesley RC, Froelicher VF. Ventricular tachycardia during routine treadmill testing. Risk and prognosis. Arch Intern Med 1991;151:349–53.

70. Marine JE, Shetty V, Chow GV, et al. Prevalence and prognostic significance of exercise-induced nonsustained ventricular tachycardia in asymptomatic volunteers. J Am Coll Cardiol 2013;62:595–600.

Outflow Tract Premature Ventricular Contractions and Ventricular Tachycardia
The Typical and the Challenging

Roy M. John, MBBS, MD, PhD*, William G. Stevenson, MD

KEYWORDS

- Outflow tract • Premature ventricular contraction • Ventricular arrhythmia • Catheter ablation

KEY POINTS

- The ventricular outflow tracts are the most common sites of origin of idiopathic ventricular arrhythmias (VAs).
- Structural heart disease should be excluded because the outflow tract can be a source of VAs in early cardiomyopathies.
- Electrocardiogram of the VA is useful in predicting potential ablation sites but careful and sequential mapping of the various structures in the outflow tract is often essential to define sites for successful ablation.
- Ablation for VAs from the right ventricular outflow tract has the highest success, followed by sites in the aortic root, left ventricular (LV) endocardium, and LV epicardium.
- The LV summit is a difficult area to access and, if catheter ablation from surrounding areas proves unsuccessful, surgical ablation is an option.

INTRODUCTION

The ventricular outflow tract is a common site of origin for premature ventricular contractions (PVCs) and repetitive ventricular tachycardia (VT) in patients with structurally normal hearts.[1] However, these sites also generate PVCs in patients with structural heart disease that tend to worsen left ventricular (LV) dysfunction. Rarely, arrhythmias from the outflow tract location can be the early manifestation of a cardiomyopathy, such as sarcoidosis, arrhythmogenic right ventricular cardiomyopathy, or acute myocarditis. Exclusion of significant disease may require the use of sophisticated imaging techniques such as cardiac MRI or PET to exclude areas of scar or inflammation that may not be evident by echocardiography.

β-Blockers and calcium channel blockers have only a modest effect in suppressing idiopathic ventricular arrhythmias (VAs), but are commonly used because of their safety. More potent antiarrhythmic drugs, such as flecainide, mexiletine, and amiodarone, are more effective but long-term use is limited by side effects. Flecainide is avoided in the presence of heart disease or depressed ventricular function. Hence, catheter ablation is an attractive option for many patients. A recent randomized study of patients with frequent PVCs from the right ventricular outflow tract (RVOT) found a greater decrease in burden of PVCs following ablation compared with drug therapy, although LV function improved in both groups.[2] However, catheter ablation for outflow tract arrhythmias is not always successful, largely

Department of Medicine, Brigham and Women's Hospital, Harvard Medical School, Boston, MA, USA
* Corresponding author. Cardiac Arrhythmia Service, Brigham and Women's Hospital, 75 Francis Street, Boston, MA 02115.
E-mail address: rjohn2@partners.org

Card Electrophysiol Clin 8 (2016) 545–554
http://dx.doi.org/10.1016/j.ccep.2016.04.004
1877-9182/16/$ – see front matter © 2016 Elsevier Inc. All rights reserved.

because of anatomic obstacles related to the three-dimensional relationship of the great vessels and their connections to the ventricular muscle. Success rates for catheter ablation largely depend on the sites of origin of these arrhythmias and their accessibility. This article reviews the relevant anatomy of the ventricular outflow regions and proximal great vessels, electrocardiographic clues to the sites of origin, and techniques commonly used to target these arrhythmias for ablation.

ANATOMY OF THE OUTFLOW TRACT

The right ventricle is a conical structure with an inlet, apical trabecular portion, and the outlet tract. The RVOT can be anatomically divided into the rightward (free wall), and leftward (septal and posterior) portions based on its relationship to the aortic root and valve, which are situated posterior and inferior to the pulmonary valve (**Fig. 1**).[3] Because the pulmonary valve is superior to and leftward of the aortic valve, the posterior-septal RVOT is closely related to the right coronary cusp (RCC) and left coronary cusp (LCC) of the aortic valve. The left main coronary artery arises from the LCC in close relationship to the posterior RVOT below the pulmonary valve. In one study, the left main coursed within 2 mm of the left pulmonary cusp in 43% of cases.[4] Although there is a theoretic risk of damage to coronary arteries from ablation in the region, none have been recorded to date, possibly because of the high flow in the coronary vessels acting as a convective coolant.

The inferior and rightward portion of the RVOT is continuous with the interventricular septum and the tricuspid annulus where the His bundle is located. In the LV outflow tract (LVOT), the RCC

and LCC lie superior to the muscular LVOT, whereas the noncoronary cusp (NCC) abuts the membranous septum and the interatrial septum (see **Fig. 1**). The NCC and the posterior aspect of the LCC are continuous with the fibrotic aortomitral continuity in the posterior-lateral aspect of the LVOT. Ventricular myocardium extends between the scallops of the semilunar valves into the both the aortic and pulmonary valves (**Fig. 2**).[5] An autopsy study showed that extensions in the LVOT are more common in the region of the RCC (55%) compared with the LCC (24%). Ventricular myocardial extension to the NCC is rare (<1%); in this region, extension of the atrial muscle is more common. In contrast, myocardial extensions above the pulmonic valves are more common and evenly distributed, occurring in 60% to 90% of patients.[6,7]

The Epicardial Outflow Tract

Idiopathic VTs are known to originate from the epicardium, usually in close relation to the venous structures.[8,9] The great cardiac vein (GCV) and its distal anterior interventricular branch can be sites for mapping and ablation of idiopathic VT.[9,10] Because the vein in this location lacks significant muscular layers (unlike the proximal course of the coronary sinus from its ostium to the valve of Vieussens), the likely origin of the VT successfully ablated from within these veins is the adjacent epicardium.

An area of interest for epicardial VTs is the LV summit, an epicardial region overlying the LV base that is anatomically defined by the region between the bifurcation of the left main coronary artery between the left anterior descending artery and left circumflex artery (**Fig. 3**).[11,12] The first septal branch defines the inferior boundary of the

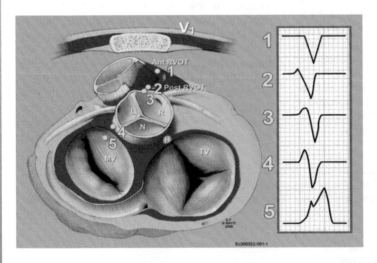

Fig. 1. The base of the left ventricle and RVOT showing leftward location of the right ventricular outflow anterior to the aortic root. QRS configuration lead V is shown for the anterior RVOT (1), posterior RVOT (2), right coronary cusp (3), left coronary cusp (4), and the region of the aortomitral continuity (5). L, left coronary cusp; MV, mitral valve; N, noncoronary cusp; R, right coronary cusp; TV, tricuspid valve. (*Adapted from* Asirvatham SJ. Correlative anatomy for the invasive electrophysiologist: outflow tract supravalvar arrhythmia. J Cardiovasc Electrophysiol 2009;20:955–68; with permission.)

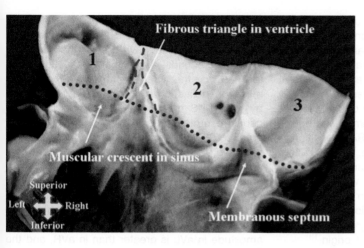

Fig. 2. Anatomic specimen showing the left ventriculoatrial junction. The aortic root has been opened from behind and spread apart. The aortic valve leaflets have been removed, revealing the semilunar nature of their attachments. The purple dotted line shows the anatomic ventriculoaortic junction, which is the union between the ventricular musculature and the aortic wall at the bases of the left and right coronary aortic valvar sinuses (*1, 2*), but between the aortic wall and fibrous continuity with the mitral valve at the base of the non-coronary sinus (*3*). Note how the semilunar attachments incorporate muscle at the base of the coronary aortic sinuses, but incorporate fibrous tissue within the ventricle as the hinge lines extend distally to reach the sinotubular junction (*red dashed triangle*). (*From* Anderson RH. The surgical anatomy of the aortic root. Multimed Man Cardiothorac Surg 2007;2007:mmcts.2006.002527; with permission.)

triangle that forms the LV summit. The GCV divides this summit region to an area above the course of the GCV where the main coronary vessels and epicardial fat make the underlying myocardium inaccessible to percutaneous catheter ablation. The region inferior to the GCV is accessible to ablation but proximity to the diagonal/intermediate coronary arteries and inability to maneuver an ablation catheter into the anterior interventricular branch (AIV) often precludes adequate ablation in the region because of the risk of coronary injury.

ELECTROCARDIOGRAM LOCALIZATION OF ORIGIN OF OUTFLOW TRACT ARRHYTHMIAS

Although the 12-lead electrocardiogram (ECG) can be helpful in the localizing site of arrhythmia origin, the complex anatomy of the outflow tract and variable distance of myocardial extensions above the valves precludes precise localization from ECG criteria alone. Systematic mapping of the RVOT, pulmonary artery, great cardiac/anterior interventricular vein via the coronary sinus, the aortic root and cusps, and LVOT is often required. In general,

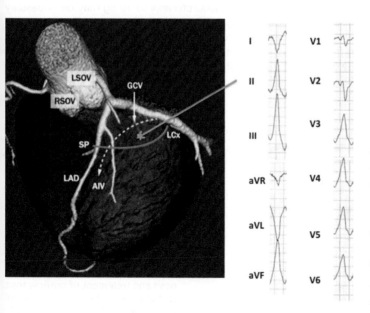

Fig. 3. The LV summit. The summit is a triangular area bounded by the bifurcation of the left main coronary artery; the inferior margin is an arbitrary line from the first septal branch (*green line*). The area is divided into superior and medial portions above the course of the GCV and the region inferior and lateral to the GCV (see text for details). A 12-lead ECG morphology of a VT arising from the accessible zone (*blue arrow*) is shown on the right. AIV, anterior interventricular branch; LAD, left anterior descending artery; LCx, left circumflex artery; LSOV, left sinus of Valsalva; RSOV, right sinus of Valsalva; SP, septal branch. (*Adapted from* Lerman BB. Mechanism, diagnosis and treatment of outflow tract tachycardia. Nat Rev Cardiol 2015; 12:596–608; with permission.)

most PVCs or VTs with left bundle branch morphology with precordial transition (the first precordial lead with R/S ratio >1) no earlier than lead V_3 and inferiorly directed axis, have an RVOT origin. A prominent R wave in V_1 or early transition before V_3 with inferior axis suggests an LVOT origin. To account for clockwise or counterclockwise rotation of the heart, algorithms have been developed comparing precordial R/S transitions during sinus rhythm with arrhythmia.[13] In LVOT arrhythmias, precordial transition occurs in the same or earlier leads than in sinus rhythm, whereas it occurs later in RVOT arrhythmia. When transition occurs in V3, an R wave transition ratio is calculated as $(R/R + S)_{VT}/(R/R + S)_{SR}$. A ratio greater than 0.6 had a high predictive value for LVOT origin.[13]

QRS complexes that are monophasic R waves without notching in leads II and III and with a duration less than 140 milliseconds usually suggest origins near the septum anterior to the aortic root, whereas an RVOT free-wall origin is suggested by a wider QRS with notching or RR' or Rr' QRS configurations in the inferior leads. For LVOT VTs, the absence of an S wave in leads V5 or V6 suggests a supravalvar location; their presence indicates an infravalvar site of origin. An aortic cusp origin is suggested by a longer duration of the R wave in leads V1 and V2 (R/QRS duration >50%) (**Fig. 4**). LCC PVCs typically display a W pattern or notching in the V1 because of early depolarization of the LV and transseptal activation.[14,15] Note that VTs originating from the aortic cusps might show preferential conduction to the RVOT, rendering these ECG criteria less reliable. In one study, 20% of VTs originating in the aortic cusps showed late QRS transition after V3.[16] Variations in the coupling intervals of PVCs may also be useful in predicting origin. PVCs emanating from the aortic root and GCV locations tend to have variations in coupling interval that exceed 60 milliseconds.[17]

Epicardial origins are suggested by delayed upstroke of the precordial QRS. Initial QRS slurring with a pseudo–delta wave greater than or equal to 34 milliseconds, a maximum deflection index (defined as the interval from QRS onset to maximum deflection in any precordial lead divided by total QRS duration measured from simultaneous recordings of all 12 leads) greater than or equal to 0.55 also suggests that epicardial mapping and ablation may be needed.[10,18] However, aortic cusp VTs can produce similar configurations.[16] Arrhythmia originating from the inferior segment of the LV summit (inferior and lateral to the GCV; see **Fig. 3**), generally have a right bundle branch block (RBBB) configuration in V1, Q-wave amplitude in aVL is greater than in aVR, and the R wave in lead III is larger than in lead II.[11]

ELECTROPHYSIOLOGIC TESTING AND MAPPING

Inability to induce the arrhythmia for mapping is one of the most common causes of ablation failure. To avoid suppression of arrhythmias, antiarrhythmic drugs should be discontinued for 5 half-lives before the procedure. In the electrophysiology laboratory, the authors place ECG leads on arrival before any sedation and record any spontaneous arrhythmia in an effort to document the 12-lead morphology. Lidocaine for local anesthesia is limited to the minimum to prevent suppression of PVCs by absorbed lidocaine. In the absence of spontaneous arrhythmia, aggressive provocation with isoproterenol, epinephrine, or atropine with or without burst pacing is used. Occasionally, boluses of isoproterenol to 40 μg may be necessary to induce idiopathic outflow tract VT. Arrhythmias tend to emerge during the washout phase of isoproterenol. Occasionally a combination of isoproterenol, atropine, and aminophylline may prove effective. Burst pacing is often more

PVC from LCC 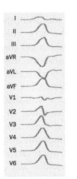 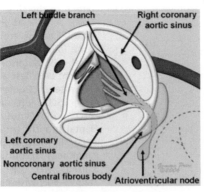 PVC from RCC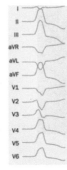

Fig. 4. Anatomy of the aortic root showing cusps, origin of the coronary arteries, and the relative position of the conduction system in relation to the cusps. Typical ECG morphologies are shown for PVCs arising from the LCC and RCC regions. (*Adapted from* Anderson RH. The surgical anatomy of the aortic root. Multimed Man Cardiothorac Surg 2007;2007:mmcts.2006.002527; and Lerman BB. Mechanism, diagnosis and treatment of outflow tract tachycardia. Nat Rev Cardiol 2015;12:596–608; with permission.)

effective than programmed stimulation. Occasionally, atrial pacing can be successful in reproducibly inducing monomorphic PVCs or nonsustained VT.

Unless the ECGs characteristics are clearly suggestive of a RVOT arrhythmia, preparations for detailed mapping with the use of an electroanatomic mapping system, intracardiac echocardiography (ICE), coronary angiography, and potential epicardial access may be necessary (**Fig. 5**). In our laboratory, we begin with systematic mapping starting with the RVOT, and progress sequentially to the GCV, aortic root, and LVOT, including the aortomitral continuity, and in selected cases the epicardium based on clues from the ECG. Combined bipolar and unipolar recordings are used for mapping the earliest activation sites. At the site of origin, bipolar recording typically precedes QRS onset by 30 milliseconds or more. The corresponding unipolar signal includes a QS complex with the earliest rapid negative deflection coinciding with the onset of the bipolar electrogram. Activation mapping is preferred to pace mapping because the latter has limited spatial resolution. Exact pace maps may be recorded up to 2 cm from the site of origin in 20% of patients.[19] In addition, preferential conduction, especially from the aortic sinuses, can render pace maps misleading. Nevertheless, pace maps may be the only means of determining approximate locations for ablation when spontaneous arrhythmias are absent or noninducible.

ABLATION OF OUTFLOW TRACT VENTRICULAR ARRHYTHMIAS
Right Ventricular Outflow Tract

Most idiopathic outflow tract arrhythmias originate in the RVOT. The commonest site of origin is in the posterior RVOT adjacent to the pulmonary valve annulus. Approximately 10% originate in the anterior free wall of the RVOT. Using intracardiac echocardiography to define the plane of the pulmonary valve, Liu and colleagues[7] showed extensions of myocardial sleeve (based on pace capture) 5 to 7 mm above the pulmonary valve in 90% of patients. Forty-six percent of RVOT arrhythmogenic foci were ablated at a median distance of 8.2 mm above the valve. These findings are intriguing and may relate to the fact that, before the common use of intracardiac echocardiography, determination of the pulmonary valve plane was based on fluoroscopy and the detection of electrograms. It is possible that the valve is frequently assigned a more superior location than its actual location and that a larger percentage of the RVOT arrhythmias are of pulmonary arterial origin. Regardless, ablation of RVOT VT based on activation and pace mapping has the highest success rate among the outflow tract arrhythmias. Local activation at successful ablation sites in the RVOT is usually 30 milliseconds presystolic. In some cases, ablation may have to be targeted at the pulmonary valve cusps, similar to aortic root arrhythmias.[20,21] In these locations, a discrete late potential is often evident during sinus rhythm that becomes the early potential during PVC or VT, suggesting a muscle strand connecting to the right ventricular musculature just as in the aortic cusps. These early potentials are usually 40 to 50 milliseconds presystolic and followed by an isoelectric period before the far-field ventricular potential. If the pulmonary valve cusp has to be targeted, it can be engaged retrograde by passing the ablation catheter through the pulmonary valve, deflecting

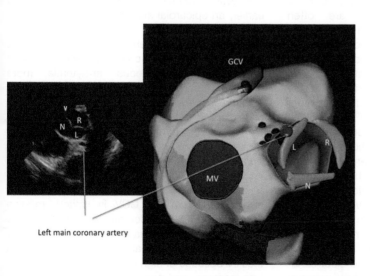

Left main coronary artery

Fig. 5. Ablation of an idiopathic VT focus with earliest activation in the GCV. A short-axis intracardiac echocardiographic view obtained with the probe position in the RVOT shows the aortic cusps and left main coronary artery origin (*left panel*). The aortic cusps and position of the left main coronary artery (*pink dots*) are marked on the electroanatomic map (*right panel*). Earliest activation (*red areas*) of an incessant slow idiopathic VT was mapped to the GCV. Radiofrequency ablations were delivered sequentially from the GCV and the LVOT below the left coronary cusps (*dark red dots*) to abolish tachycardia that had its origin deep within the myocardium.

and withdrawing into the respective pulmonary cusp.

Even for the seemingly straightforward RVOT arrhythmias, a recent multicenter study showed an 18% recurrence rate during long-term follow-up, reflecting the difficulties in precise localization and durable ablation of arrhythmias from the outflow tract.[22] A common cause for failed ablation for an apparent RVOT arrhythmia is the reluctance to investigate the potential origin of the arrhythmia in the aortic root that is positioned immediately posterior to the posterior aspect of the RVOT and where arrhythmias may have ECG features that mimic an RVOT origin (discussed earlier).

Aortic Root

The most common site of origin of LVOT ventricular arrhythmia is the aortic root or cusps. The region around the LCC is the most frequent site, followed by the RCC-LCC commissure, the RCC, and rarely the NCC.[20] Catheter manipulation in the aortic sinuses can be challenging and ICE is helpful in visualizing the aortic cusps (see **Fig. 5**) and the coronary ostia, and in locating the catheter in the region of the cusps. Detailed mapping is important to avoid missing small local potentials that often precede far-field potentials from the ventricular myocardium. A discrete potential is detectable in up to 25% of patients from the regions of the LCC and RCC.[23] They may be seen as late potentials during sinus rhythm. During PVC or VT, this potential is often followed by an isoelectric period of 40 milliseconds or more before the far-field local ventricular electrogram that corresponds with the surface QRS and QS wave on unipolar recording. Attempts to pace capture the discrete potential are often confounded by far-field capture and a misleading pace map that does not look like the arrhythmia.[16,24] The discrete potentials are thought to emanate from an insulated strand of muscle fiber that connects to ventricular muscle in the RVOT, subvalvar LV myocardium, or other areas of the aortic root, resulting in activation distant from the origin.[24] Ablation along the course of the fiber can result in elimination, delay, or dissociation of the discrete potential in sinus rhythm with successful abolition of the arrhythmia. When discrete potentials are not evident, ablation in the area immediately below the valve plane to target the insertion site can often be successful.

Safe ablation in the aortic sinus requires clear definition of the origin of the main coronary arteries. The combined use of ICE and electroanatomic mapping allows for tagging of the origin of the vessels and monitoring to ensure a safe distance during ablation (see **Fig. 5**). However, most of the sites for ablation are well below the coronary orifices. Occasionally, coronary angiography is necessary. For ablations in the aortic root, nonirrigation catheters provide sufficient energy for localized lesions to render the tissue nonexcitable. However, to avoid potential thrombus formation, the authors tend to use an irrigated catheter and gradually titrate power, starting at 10 W and increasing to a maximum of 30 W, aiming for an impedance drop of 10 Ω.

Aortomitral Continuity

Idiopathic VT may originate from regions around the mitral annulus and display an inferior axis when the region of the aortomitral continuity and left fibrous trigone is involved. Typically, VT has an RBBB configuration (a qR pattern may be present in V1) with S waves in V6.[25] A retrograde aortic or transseptal approach to the region allows adequate catheter contact for effective ablation.

Epicardial and Perivenous Foci

Between 2.5% and 15% of idiopathic VAs originate from the epicardial LV. Regions where these arrhythmias are successfully ablated segregate to the area of the GCV, the myocardium underlying the AIV branch, and at the crux of the heart accessible via the middle cardiac vein. The LV summit superior and inferior to the distal GCV is the most common site for these arrhythmias (see **Fig. 3**). Because the site of successful ablation does not necessarily correspond with sites of origin of the arrhythmia, the exact foci of origin of these arrhythmias is not clearly defined.

In addition to clues from the ECG, as described earlier, an epicardial source for the arrhythmia is suggested by earliest activation in the GCV compared with any endocardial site. Further, pace maps from the coronary venous system approximate spontaneous arrhythmia more closely compared with endocardial sites. Before ablation is performed, coronary angiography is necessary to ensure adequate distance of the catheter tip (>5 mm) from an epicardial coronary vessel to prevent injury. In more lateral locations, phrenic nerve capture should be tested with pacing to avoid the possibility of phrenic nerve damage. Success for abolition of epicardial arrhythmias from the GCV is limited, ranging from 50% to 70%.[8,26] Common reasons for failure include the inability to maneuver a catheter distally into the GCV and AIV, inability to delivery energy in the AIV because of high impedance and temperature increase, and proximity to coronary vessels.

When ablation in the GCV/AIV is precluded, alternative sites to be considered for ablation include the left sinus of Valsalva, the closest endocardial site opposite the GCV/AIV (including the aortomitral continuity), and the most leftward aspect of the posterior RVOT that closely overlies the AIV.[26–28] Despite fairly late activation (<10 milliseconds) and poor pace maps, ablation in these locations can be successful in some patients. In one study, successful ablation from the left sinus of Valsalva or adjacent LV endocardium was predicted when the anatomic distance between them and the GCV/AIV was less than 13.5 mm and the ECG of the arrhythmia showed a Q-wave ratio in aVL/aVR of less than 1.45.[28] If these attempts fail, percutaneous epicardial mapping is a consideration.

THE CHALLENGING CASES

Although idiopathic PVCs or repetitive VT have a generally good prognosis, the occasional patient with incessant and/or highly symptomatic arrhythmia or arrhythmia-induced LV dysfunction warrants aggressive steps to suppress the arrhythmia. Ablation becomes challenging when the early activation is not identified in the RVOT or aortic cusps. It is worth emphasizing that detection of an early potential in the aortic sinus requires meticulous high-resolution mapping, and the presence of electrical noise can easily obscure small signals. A systematic approach to mapping both outflow tracts, the epicardial venous system, and in some cases the epicardium is usually successful in identifying the arrhythmia locations for ablation.

The most difficult arrhythmia foci for ablation are those that are mapped to the LV summit. Ablation in the area of the summit superior and medial to the GCV is often precluded by the presence of the bifurcation of the left coronary artery. Most of the arrhythmias in this location have an intramural origin between the epicardial LV summit and the endocardial aortomitral continuity or basal septum. An intramural location is suggested by activation times less than 10 milliseconds pre-QRS from both epicardial and endocardial locations and the far-field (rounded signals with low dV/dT) nature of early electrograms. Pace maps are more likely to approximate the spontaneous arrhythmia when high output is used compared with low-output pacing, which is likely only to capture the local myocardial surface. In addition, it is common to see late and transient suppression of arrhythmia during ablation. Dual-site simultaneous unipolar ablation with radiofrequency energy can be effective even when the distance separating the ablation sites is more than 8 mm.[29] For distances less than 8 mm, sequential ablations from the opposing surfaces can be effective.

When percutaneous, catheter-based mapping and ablation prove unsuccessful, surgical ablation is a consideration. Minimally invasive and open surgical approaches have been described for surgical cryoablation of epicardial VT from the LV summit.[30,31] Deep general anesthesia tends to suppress spontaneous arrhythmia and pace mapping can be difficult because of chest retraction changing the anatomic relationship to the heart. The use of radiographic markers such as a pacing lead in the AIV can be useful in identification of sites of earliest activation on the epicardium (**Fig. 6**). Under direct vision, the main coronary arteries can be mobilized in slings to allow application of cryoablation to the myocardium deep to the vessels. Surgical cryoablation can be successful in arrhythmia suppression but coronary injury with late stenosis remains a risk.[30]

OUTCOMES AND COMPLICATIONS OF CATHETER ABLATION FOR OUTFLOW TRACT ARRHYTHMIAS

Despite mounting enthusiasm for ablation for idiopathic PVCs, success defined as at least an 80% reduction in ectopic activity is lower than previously published. In a recent multicenter retrospective analysis of 1185 patients undergoing ablations at 8 specialized centers, acute overall procedural success was 84%. However, when these patients were followed with postprocedure Holter monitor, success rate without antiarrhythmic drugs was 71%.[22] Predictors of success were RVOT origin (82% success), a nonepicardial focus, and absence of multiple morphologies. Repeat procedures were required in 22%, most commonly for arrhythmias of epicardial origin that required a mean of 1.6 procedures. Another common reason for failure is the inability to induce the arrhythmia for adequate mapping.[32]

The most common complications relate to vascular access (2.8%). Pericardial tamponade occurs in less than 1% of cases and is most common with ablation for an epicardial focus.[22] Damage to the epicardial coronary arteries can occur with ablation in the epicardial venous system. Risk can be minimized by keeping a minimum distance of 5 mm from a coronary vessel or by the use of cryoablation. In the posterior RVOT, power is probably best limited to 30 W to prevent collateral damage, especially in young patients. Atrioventricular block is a risk for ablation of foci adjacent to the conduction system.

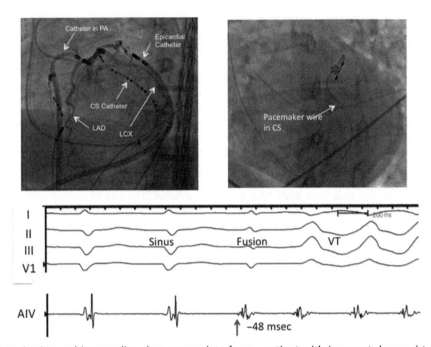

Fig. 6. Catheterization and intracardiac electrogram data from a patient with incessant drug-resistant VT from the LV summit. Left coronary angiography and multipolar mapping catheters (*top left panel*) and a fluoroscopic image in left anterior oblique view of a pacing lead in the AIV branch of the coronary sinus (*top right panel*) are shown. Earliest activation was seen in the GCV but a bipolar pacing lead inserted over a guidewire to the proximal anterior interventricular branch registered the earliest activation (−48 milliseconds pre-QRS), marked by red asterisks in the top panels and a red arrow in the bottom panel. The earliest site was too close to the first diagonal branch for epicardial catheter ablation. The patient underwent successful surgical cryoablation with the pacing lead acting as a fluoroscopic marker in the operating room, where arrhythmia could not be induced under deep anesthesia. PA, pulmonary artery. (*Adapted from* Choi EK, Nagashima K, Lin KY, et al. Surgical cryoablation for ventricular tachyarrhythmia arising from the left ventricular outflow tract region. Heart Rhythm 2015;12:1128–36; with permission.)

SUMMARY

In recent years, significant advances have occurred in the understanding of idiopathic ventricular arrhythmia sources from the outflow tract. Most arrhythmias can be safely ablated in the RVOT or aortic cusps but some require more detailed and meticulous mapping in the epicardium via the venous system. The use of ICE and electroanatomic mapping systems is critical to successful ablation in non-RVOT locations. Although the surface ECG of the arrhythmia offers important clues, systematic mapping of all potential locations to define origins can improve success rates. In the rare cases in which catheter-based ablation is precluded or unsuccessful because of locations in the LV summit, surgical ablation remains an option.

REFERENCES

1. Miles WM. Idiopathic ventricular outflow tract tachycardia: where does it originate? J Cardiovasc Electrophysiol 2001;12:536–7.

2. Ling Z, Liu Z, Su L, et al. Radiofrequency ablation vs. antiarrhythmic medication for treatment of ventricular premature beats from the right ventricular outflow tract: a prospective randomized study. Circ Arrhythm Electrophysiol 2014;7:237–43.

3. Asirvatham SJ. Correlative anatomy for the invasive electrophysiologist: outflow tract supravalvar arrhythmia. J Cardiovasc Electrophysiol 2009;20:955–68.

4. Walsh KA, Fahey GJ. Anatomy of the left main coronary artery of particular relevance to ablation of left atrial and outflow tract arrhythmias. Heart Rhythm 2014;11:2231–8.

5. Anderson RH. The surgical anatomy of the aortic root. Multimed Man Cardiothorac Surg 2007;2007. mmcts.2006.002527.

6. Gami AS, Noheria A, Lachman N, et al. Anatomical correlates relevant to ablation above the semilunar valves for the cardiac electrophysiologist: a study of 603 hearts. J Interv Card Electrophysiol 2011;30:5–15.

7. Liu CF, Cheung JW, Thomas G, et al. Ubiquitous myocardial extensions into the pulmonary artery

demonstrated by integrated intracardiac echocardiography and electroanatomic mapping: changing the paradigm of idiopathic right ventricular outflow tract arrhythmias. Circ Arrhythm Electrophysiol 2014;7:691–700.

8. Baman TS, Ilg KJ, Gupta SK, et al. Mapping and ablation of epicardial idiopathic ventricular arrhythmias from within the coronary venous system. Circ Arrhythm Electrophysiol 2010;3:274–9.

9. Li YC, Lin JF, Li J, et al. Catheter ablation of idiopathic ventricular arrhythmias originating from the left ventricular epicardium adjacent to the transitional area of the great cardiac vein to the anterior interventricular vein. Int J Cardiol 2013;167: 2673–81.

10. Daniels DV, Lu YY, Morton JB, et al. Idiopathic epicardial left ventricular tachycardia originating remote from the sinus of Valsalva: electrophysiological characteristics, catheter ablation, and identification from the 12-lead electrocardiogram. Circulation 2006;113:1659–66.

11. Yamada T, McElderry HT, Doppalapudi H, et al. Idiopathic ventricular arrhythmias originating from the left ventricular summit: anatomic concepts relevant to ablation. Circ Arrhythm Electrophysiol 2010;3: 616–23.

12. Lerman BB. Mechanism, diagnosis and treatment of outflow tract tachycardia. Nat Rev Cardiol 2015;12: 597–608.

13. Betensky BP, Park RE, Marchlinski FE, et al. The V_2 transition ratio: a new electrocardiographic criterion for distinguishing left from right ventricular outflow tract tachycardia origin. J Am Coll Cardiol 2011;57: 2255–62.

14. Ouyang F, Fotuhi P, Ho SY, et al. Repetitive monomorphic ventricular tachycardia originating from the aortic sinus cusp: electrocardiographic characterization for guiding catheter ablation. J Am Coll Cardiol 2002;39:500–8.

15. Hachiya H, Aonuma K, Yamauchi Y, et al. How to diagnose, locate and ablate coronary cusp ventricular tachycardia. J Cardiovasc Electrophysiol 2002;13: 551–6.

16. Yamada T, Murakami Y, Yoshida N, et al. Preferential conduction across the ventricular outflow septum in ventricular arrhythmias originating from the aortic sinus cusp. J Am Coll Cardiol 2007; 50(9):884–91.

17. Bradfield JS, Homsi M, Shivkumar K, et al. Coupling interval variability differentiates ventricular ectopic complexes arising in the aortic sinus of Valsalva and great cardiac vein from other sources: mechanistic and arrhythmic risk implications. J Am Coll Cardiol 2014;63(20):2151–8.

18. Berruezo A, Mont L, Nava S, et al. Electrocardiographic recognition of the epicardial origins of ventricular tachycardias. Circulation 2004;109:1842–7.

19. Bogun F, Tai M, Kim HM, et al. Spatial resolution of pacemapping of idiopathic ventricular tachycardia/ectopy originating in the right ventricular outflow tract. Heart Rhythm 2008;5:339–44.

20. Timmermans C, Rodriguez LM, Medeiros A, et al. Radiofrequency catheter ablation of idiopathic ventricular tachycardia originating in the main stem of the pulmonary artery. J Cardiovasc Electrophysiol 2002;13:281–4.

21. Liao Z, Zhan X, Wu S, et al. Idiopathic ventricular arrhythmia originating from the pulmonary sinus cusp. Prevalence, electrocardiographic/electrophysiological characteristics and catheter ablation. J Am Coll Cardiol 2015;66:2613–44.

22. Latchamsetty R, Yokokawa M, Morady F, et al. Multicenter outcomes for catheter ablation of idiopathic premature ventricular complexes. JACCCEP 2015; 1(3):116–23.

23. Yamada T, McElderry T, Doppalpudi H, et al. Idiopathic ventricular arrhythmia originating from the aortic root: prevalence, electrocardiographic and electrophysiologic characteristics and results of radiofrequency catheter ablation. J Am Coll Cardiol 2008;52:139–47.

24. Hachiya H, Yamauchi Y, Iesaka Y, et al. Discrete prepotentials as an indicator of successful ablation in patients with coronary cusp ventricular arrhythmia. Circ Arrhythm Electrophysiol 2013;6: 898–904.

25. Chen J, Hoff PI, Rossvoll O, et al. Ventricular arrhythmias origination from the aortomitral continuity: an uncommon variant of the left ventricular outflow tract tachycardia. Europace 2012;14:388–95.

26. Nagashima K, Choi EK, Lin KY, et al. Ventricular arrhythmias near the distal great cardiac vein: challenging arrhythmia for ablation. Circ Arrhythm Electrophysiol 2014;7:906–12.

27. Frankel D, Mountantonakis SE, Dahu MI, et al. Elimination of ventricular arrhythmias originating from the anterior interventricular vein with ablation in the right ventricular outflow tract. Circ Arrhythm Electrophysiol 2014;7:984–5.

28. Jauregui Abularach ME, Campos B, Park KM, et al. Ablation of ventricular arrhythmias arising near the anterior epicardial veins from the left sinus of Valsalva region: ECG features, anatomic distance, and outcome. Heart Rhythm 2012;9:865–73.

29. Yamada T, Maddox WR, McElederry T, et al. Radiofrequency catheter ablation of idiopathic ventricular arrhythmias originating from intramural foci in the left ventricular outflow tract: efficacy of sequential versus simultaneous unipolar catheter ablation. Circ Arrhythm Electrophysiol 2015;8:344–52.

30. Choi EK, Nagashima K, Lin KY, et al. Surgical cryoablation for ventricular tachyarrhythmia arising from the left ventricular outflow tract region. Heart Rhythm 2015;12:1128–36.

31. Mulpuru SK, Feld GK, Madani M, et al. A novel minimally-invasive surgical approach for ablation of ventricular tachycardia originating near the proximal left anterior descending artery. Circ Arrhythm Electrophysiol 2012;5:e95–7.

32. Choi EK, Kumar S, Nagashimi K, et al. Better outcome of ablation for sustained outflow-tract ventricular tachycardia when tachycardia is inducible. Europace 2015. http://dx.doi.org/10.1093/europace/euv064.

Spectrum of Ventricular Arrhythmias Arising from Papillary Muscle in the Structurally Normal Heart

Niyada Naksuk, MD[a], Suraj Kapa, MD[a],
Samuel J. Asirvatham, MD[a,b],*

KEYWORDS

- Papillary arrhythmias • Papillary muscle • Premature ventricular contraction
- Structurally normal heart • Ventricular arrhythmias • Ventricular fibrillation • Ventricular tachycardia

KEY POINTS

- Ventricular arrhythmias arising from the papillary muscle account for 4% to 12% of arrhythmias in a structurally normal heart and are generally non–life threatening.
- Although distinguishing arrhythmias from papillary muscle and Purkinje tissue is challenging, an attempt should be made because the techniques used in ablation are different.
- Ablation assisted by real-time imaging modalities still has a variable success rate.
- Malignant arrhythmias related to the papillary muscle may be secondary to focal ectopy triggering ventricular fibrillation.

 Video content accompanies this article at http://www.cardiacep.theclinics.com.

INTRODUCTION

Papillary muscles are endocardial structures that can harbor arrhythmic substrate in structural heart disease and an apparently normal heart.[1,2] In patients without a prior infarct, papillary muscles account for 4% to 12% of idiopathic ventricular arrhythmias.[3,4] Both the right and left papillary muscles can be arrhythmogenic, although reported cases involving right ventricular (RV) papillary muscles are scarce. Because of the anatomic complex of the papillary muscles, differentiating with other arrhythmias arising from adjacent/close by structures is challenging. In particular, distinguishing myocardial versus fascicular origin is essentially impossible given their close anatomic relationship. However, it is worth attempting because different techniques for ablation of papillary arrhythmias are required and potential complications after ablation may be different between these two entities. Catheter ablation has a fair success rate because of the difficulty in maintaining catheter stability, the thickness of muscle, and its complex anatomy. Published studies regarding approaches for ablation are limited because of its relative rarity.

Financial Support: None.
The authors have nothing to disclose.
[a] Division of Cardiovascular Diseases, Department of Medicine, Mayo Clinic, 200 First Street Southwest, Rochester, MN 55905, USA; [b] Division of Pediatric Cardiology, Department of Pediatric and Adolescent Medicine, Mayo Clinic, 200 First Street Southwest, Rochester, MN 55905, USA
* Corresponding author. Division of Cardiovascular Diseases, Department of Pediatrics and Adolescent Medicine, Mayo Clinic, 200 First Street Southwest, Rochester, MN 55905.
E-mail address: asirvatham.samuel@mayo.edu

Card Electrophysiol Clin 8 (2016) 555–565
http://dx.doi.org/10.1016/j.ccep.2016.04.005
1877-9182/16/$ – see front matter © 2016 Elsevier Inc. All rights reserved.

ANATOMIC CORRELATION AND PHYSIOLOGIC CONSIDERATION

Papillary muscles are supporting subvalvular structures of the mitral and tricuspid valves.[5] These muscles are a complex pouching of the ventricular wall that often vary in shape. Their thickness (generally equal to the left ventricular [LV] wall) results in higher energy requirement for radiofrequency ablation than the usual dose.[6]

The mitral valve usually has two associated papillary muscles (posteromedial and anterolateral), which are supplied by either the right coronary or the circumflex artery (dependent of the dominance), and dual blood supplies from the left anterior descending and the circumflex arteries, respectively. Hence, the posteromedial papillary muscle is more vulnerable to ischemic injury than the anterolateral muscle. Interestingly, even in patients without a history of infarct or structural heart disease, idiopathic ventricular tachycardia (VT) or premature ventricular contractions (PVCs) tend to originate predominantly from the posteromedial papillary muscle.[7,8]

The posteromedial papillary muscle lies in between the LV septum and posterior free wall, whereas the anterolateral papillary muscle lies on the anterolateral free wall.[7] The locations where their large bases insert the LV wall serve as an anatomic landmark for the beginning of the apical component of the LV. Two papillary muscles are located close to each other, which can cause difficulties in manipulating the catheter (**Fig. 1**). Furthermore, papillary arrhythmias may exhibit multiple QRS morphologies caused by variable exit sites from an intramural focus or its attachment to false cords.[8]

The RV papillary muscles include the anterolateral, posteromedial, and septal (or medial) muscles (**Fig. 2**). The latter seems to be the most common site for arrhythmias according to a single available study.[9] Of anatomic importance, the septal muscle arises from the RV outflow tract (RVOT), and is commonly referred to the Lancisi muscle or the conus papillary muscle.[5] Ventricular arrhythmias arising from this location may have a similar QRS complex to that of arrhythmias arising from the RVOT.[5]

The Purkinje fiber–muscular interface that exists within the papillary muscles may play an important role in the genesis of papillary muscle–related arrhythmias.[10] This close relationship between the Purkinje fiber and papillary muscles has made some difficulties to distinguish arrhythmias from the two structures. In a study of heart dissection, there is Purkinje tissue coming from the anterior fascicle at the region of the anterolateral papillary muscle and the left posterior fascicle inserts near the base of the posteromedial muscle.[11,12] The RV papillary muscles also have anatomic relationship to the cardiac conduction system. The right bundle branch becomes more superficial to the subendocardial layer at the base of the septal papillary muscle. A major fascicle of the right bundle branch continues within the moderator band that connects to the anterior papillary muscle where its Purkinje fibers spread out.[13,14]

CLINICAL MANIFESTATIONS

Idiopathic papillary ventricular arrhythmias are commonly induced by exercise and generally have a benign course.[4,8] Syncope and cardiac arrest are rare. The PVCs and nonsustained VT are more common than sustained VT. Frequent papillary PVCs can induce cardiomyopathy that is reversible if suppression of the PVCs is successful.[9] There are also reported cases of PVCs from the papillary muscle triggering VF. In patients with mitral valve prolapse (MVP), the papillary muscle has been reported to be a critical site of ventricular arrhythmias that may lead to sudden cardiac arrest.[15] Malignant arrhythmias related to the papillary muscle are discussed in a latter section.

DIFFERENTIAL DIAGNOSIS

Idiopathic LV arrhythmias arising from the papillary muscles, left fascicles, and mitral annulus, and ventricular arrhythmias arising from the conus

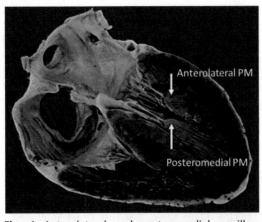

Fig. 1. Anterolateral and posteromedial papillary muscles (PM) of the left ventricle. Note their broad bases that locate close approximation to each other. (*From* Abouezzeddine O, Suleiman M, Buescher T, et al. Relevance of endocavitary structures in ablation procedures for ventricular tachycardia. J Cardiovas Electrophysiol 2010;21(3):246; with permission.)

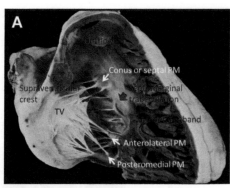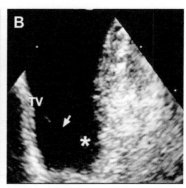

Fig. 2. (*A*) Papillary muscles of the right ventricle and their anatomic relationship to tendinous chordal connection, the tricuspid valve (TV), and the moderator band. (*B*) Intracardiac ultrasound shows the tendinous chord (*arrow*) that is part of the tricuspid valve (TV) attached to the body of the conus papillary muscle (*asterix*). (*From* Hai JJ, Desimone CV, Vaidya VR, et al. Endocavitary structures in the outflow tract: anatomy and electrophysiology of the conus papillary muscles. J Cardiovas Electrophysiol 2014;25(1):97; with permission.)

papillary muscle and RVOT, can have relatively similar QRS morphologies.[8] Integration of clinical findings, electrocardiography (ECG), and electrophysiologic study findings is essential to understanding the precise source of arrhythmias.

Electrocardiography

Patients with idiopathic papillary arrhythmias usually have normal ECGs during sinus rhythm.[4,16] Similar to other VTs originating from the LV, papillary arrhythmias have a right bundle branch morphology in lead V1. Arrhythmias from the posteromedial papillary muscle usually have a superior axis, similar to arrhythmias from the left posterior fascicle and the posterior half of the mitral annulus.[1,17] Arrhythmias from the anterolateral papillary muscle often have an inferior axis, which is similar to arrhythmias from the left anterior fascicle and the anterior half of the mitral annulus.[4,17]

Some proposed characteristics may help distinguish between these different sources of idiopathic LV arrhythmias. Generally, wider QRS complex and the absence of an rR′ pattern are often observed in papillary arrhythmias, when compared with fascicular VT.[10,17,18] An algorithm recently proposed by a study based on 18 patients with papillary arrhythmias, suggests approximately 90% sensitivity and specificity in differentiating these arrhythmias by using a QRS greater than 130 milliseconds as a cutoff.[17] When compared with mitral annular arrhythmias, papillary muscles are less likely to give a positive precordial VT.[17] It is, however, important to emphasize that there is still a great overlap between these entities, particularly papillary and Purkinje arrhythmias (**Fig. 3**).

Ventricular arrhythmias originating from the RV papillary muscles are more uncommon than those from the LV papillary muscles. However, arrhythmias from the septal papillary muscle can be confused with idiopathic arrhythmias from the RVOT, the most common VT in a structurally normal heart.[5] Some helpful ECG features were noted from limited case series.[9] Arrhythmias from the posterior or anterior RV papillary muscles more often have a superior axis with a late R-wave transition (>V4) as compared with septal papillary muscle arrhythmias, which often have an inferior axis and an earlier R-wave transition.[9] In comparison with arrhythmias from the RVOT, right-sided papillary VT typically has a wider QRS complex with a notched appearance in the precordial leads.

Imaging

Cardiac magnetic resonance (CMR) is commonly used as part of an initial work-up of patients presenting with ventricular arrhythmias; however, most idiopathic papillary arrhythmias have a normal CMR.[10] An exception was reported among those with MVP, which may be considered a form of structural heart disease. Studies have shown that late gadolinium enhancement (LGE) localized on the papillary muscles may be seen in patients with MVP with ventricular arrhythmias, but not in patients with MVP without a history of ventricular arrhythmias.[19,20] Although patients with bileaflet MVP and complex PVCs arising from both the papillary muscles and the outflow tracts were recently proposed as being at increased risk of malignant ventricular arrhythmias,[15] a direct link between the LGE of papillary muscles and malignant arrhythmias has not been confirmed in cohorts with electrophysiologic studies.

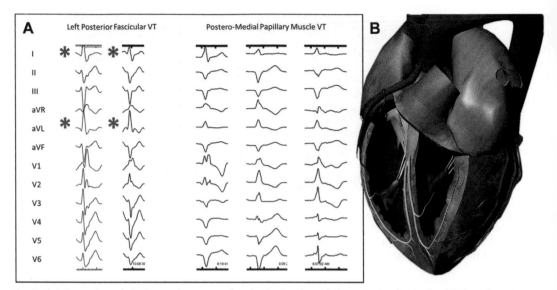

Fig. 3. (A) Examples of electrocardiograms of arrhythmias from left posterior fascicular (LPF) and posterome-dial papillary muscle (PM). Notice that the QRS width and QRS morphology in V1 are not sufficient to distin-guish the two arrhythmias. However, the presence of a q or Q wave in the lateral leads (I and VL) may discriminate the LPF from the PM ventricular tachycardia (*asterisk*). We hypothesize that the q/Q waves indicate early left-to-right septal depolarization during an LPF VT. (B) The PL papillary muscle is a slightly more lateral structure and the septal depolarization occurs later in the QRS; hence, the absence of q/Q waves in the lateral leads.

Electrophysiologic Characteristics

Idiopathic papillary VT is not typically inducible by programmed ventricular or atrial pacing, suggest-ing a nonreentrant mechanism.[4,16] A focal mecha-nism for idiopathic papillary arrhythmias is further supported by the typical lack of low voltage or fractionated potentials at the sites of ablation suc-cess, inducibility with isoproterenol or epinephrine infusion and burst pacing, and the finding that the first beat of tachycardia is typically similar to sub-sequent beats.[21]

Purkinje potentials can be found very close to the onset of QRS or slightly after the beginning of QRS complex during sinus rhythm and the targeted papillary arrhythmias in some cases (25%–45%). This may reflect a more superficial source rather than one deeper within the body of papillary muscle.[4,10,16] Ablationists therefore do not use these Purkinje signals as ablation target. In contrast, two distinct prediastolic and presystolic Purkinje potentials (ie, P1 and P2) representing macroreentrant VT can be clearly recognized in most cases during the mapping of arrhythmias (75%–100%) and any of P1 sig-nals can be targeted for successful ablation.[10,22,23]

Papillary arrhythmias can exhibit multiple QRS morphologies. Yamada and colleagues[8] found spontaneous subtle changes in the QRS during an electrophysiology study. With notion that a sin-gle wide ablation at the base of the papillary mus-cle was successful, the authors hypothesized that this was caused by multiple exits from a single intrapapillary focus.[4] Furthermore, there are many other endocavitary structures that can con-nect the papillary muscle, such as the chordae tendineae and false tendons through which con-ducting fibers can run, supporting the authors' hypothesis.[21]

TREATMENT AND PROGNOSIS

In general, idiopathic ventricular arrhythmias in a structurally normal heart including those origi-nating from papillary muscles carry an excellent prognosis. Such cases may require only follow-up even with frequent PVCs if the patient is asymp-tomatic and has a preserved LV ejection fraction.[2] Rarely, frequent ventricular ectopy (generally defined as >10,000–20,000 per 24 hours or >10%–20% of total QRS complex) can cause PVC or tachycardia-mediated cardiomyopathy in which therapy is warranted.[24] Additionally, papil-lary muscles rarely can trigger VF in a patient without known structural heart disease. Predis-posing risk factors have not been determined in such cases.

There is no consensus to date whether or which antiarrhythmic drug is most effective in papillary arrhythmias. Based on limited studies including patients with symptomatic papillary arrhythmia requiring ablation, sodium-channel blockers and verapamil are typically ineffective and thus ablation seems to be a universal approach.[4]

Catheter Ablation Techniques

Attempt to define arrhythmias arising from the papillary muscle versus Purkinje fiber is helpful in planning the ablation because of different catheter manipulation, energy delivery, and the requirement for an intracardiac ultrasound. Furthermore, avoiding extensive ablation on Purkinje fibers may be preferred because loss of the contribution of Purkinje fiber network to ventricular contraction can theoretically predispose to electrical dyssynchrony.[25]

One difficulty associated with ablation of papillary arrhythmias is maintaining contact of the ablation catheter with the contracting muscle during systole.[26] It is not clear whether transseptal or retrograde aortic approaches is better in this particular setting. Generally, transseptal mapping approach may be associated with a higher contact force, whereas the retrograde aortic approach may offer higher catheter stability in the mid- and apical-segments (where the bases of LV papillary muscles attach).[27,28] Consequently, the two techniques may complement each other and, ultimately, the approach must be tailored to the patient and operator. We note that the published data enrolling patients requiring ablation of papillary arrhythmias tended to use the retrograde aortic approach (Table 1).

Integrated intracardiac echocardiography (ICE) guided imaging with electroanatomic mapping should be used to achieve a higher success rate.[6,26,29] An ICE probe can be positioned in the RV to allow real-time and continuous monitoring and sequential acquisition of electrogram-gated images of the LV (Fig. 4).[30,31] In general for the LV papillary muscles, the anterior and posterior aspects of the anterolateral papillary muscle and the septal aspect of posteromedial papillary muscle reflect the most frequently identified arrhythmogenic site. Arrhythmias from the RV papillary muscles originate equally from the base and middle portions.[4]

Catheter ablation of papillary arrhythmias is typically performed at the site of the earliest endocardial activation. Activation mapping is the most commonly used technique.[4,8] Pace mapping is necessary when PVCs are infrequent because of its inconsistent results given that substrate is anywhere along the papillary muscle, but the pace mapping only correlates with the exit site.[16]

Furthermore, given the possibility of capturing more papillary muscle tissue beyond just the arrhythmogenic focus, pace mapping can be inaccurate or misleading. Based on activation or pace map, targeting for ablation includes the earliest prepotential bipolar activity or the presence of Purkinje potential at the site. Energies during radiofrequency ablation of 30 to 70 W have been reported to be necessary to achieve impendence drops of up to 8 to 10 Ω.[8] A relatively wide area (approximately half) of the papillary muscle's circumference and multiple ablation lesions may need to be targeted because of the potential for a deep intramural focus with multiple exits.[8] The procedure is likely successful by using an irrigated or larger tip catheter. A few studies note either an irrigated 3.5-mm tip catheter or an 8-mm tipped nonirrigated ablation catheter was likely linked to greater success rates compared with a 4-mm nonirrigated small catheter (see Table 1).[4,8,32] In our institution, we prefer an irrigated catheter, which allows the creation of larger and deeper lesion, less temperature increase, and lower local thrombus formation compared with a nonirrigated catheter.[6] Maintaining activated clotting time greater than 250 seconds with adequate anticoagulation is recommended to prevent thrombus formation during ablation.[6]

Cryoablation has been used when traditional radiofrequency ablation failed and may be effective because of improved contact stability. Accepted end points include noninducibility by isoproterenol or epinephrine infusion or burst pacing. Overall, the total number of lesions and ablation time are reportedly higher when targeting arrhythmias originating from the papillary muscles compared with other sites.[1,3]

Injury to neighboring structures particularly the atrioventricular valves is of concern. Each of the two LV papillary muscles attach to chordae tendineae supporting the anterior and posterior leaflets, thus damage to either muscle may affect both leaflets.[33] Although data from limited case series reported none of these fearful complications, avoiding excessive ablation, careful titration of power, and obtaining postoperative echocardiography are important.[4] Our group reported a successful ablation of a targeted lesion near the tip of the anterolateral papillary muscle by isolation near the base of the muscle to avoid an injury near the calcified myocardium and related chordae tendineae.[30] If this fails and the tip of the papillary muscle is certainly requiring ablation, ICE is helpful in guiding sufficient but limited ablation (Video 1).

Attention to ICE is always useful in the determination of the morphology and attachment of the papillary muscles, which may be crucial to avoid

Table 1
Published studies of left ventricular papillary muscle arrhythmias in a normally structural heart requiring ablation

Study	Study Patients	Transseptal or Retrograde Aortic Approach	Catheter	Mapping Technique	Ablation Technique	Site of Ablation	Complication	Efficacy of First Ablation (%)	Recurrences
Santoro et al,[35] 2014	5 (1 LV-PM, 4 RV-PL)	Both	A 3.5-mm open irrigated catheter	Electroanatomic mapping (Carto), pacing and activation mapping	Ablation at the earliest activation point matched pace mapping	Base of the PM papillary muscle	None	100	0% (58 mo f/u)
Yamada et al,[8] 2010	19 (7 LV-AL, 12 LV-PM)	Retrograde aortic approach	Mixed; a 3.5-mm open irrigated catheter or a nonirrigated catheter (4 or 8 mm)	Electroanatomic mapping (Carto), pacing, and activation mapping	Ablation guided by pace mapping failed to eliminate all VAs. Electroanatomic mapping exhibited a larger target.	Base of the papillary muscle	Not reported	95	58%, unknown duration
Good et al,[10] 2008	5 (4 LV-AL, 1 LV-PM)	Not reported	First attempt with a 4-mm nonirrigated catheter. If insufficient power, a 3.5-mm open irrigated catheter was used.	Electroanatomic mapping (Carto), pacing, and activation mapping	Ablation at the earliest activation during activation mapping for frequent PVCs and pacing for noninducible PVCs	Not reported	None	100	Unknown[a]

Doppalapudi et al,[16] 2008	7 (7 LV-PM)	Retrograde aortic approach	First attempt with a nonirrigated catheter (3.5 or 5 mm). Second attempts after recurrence with a 3-mm externally irrigated catheter or a 4-mm internally irrigated catheter.	Activation mapping	Ablation at the earliest site of activation mapping	Base of the PM papillary muscle	None	100	0%, unknown duration
Yokokawa et al,[26] 2010	18[b]	Not reported	First attempt with a 3.5-mm open irrigated catheter. If failed, a 6-mm cryocatheter was used.	Electroanatomic mapping (Carto), pacing, and activation mapping	Ablation at the earliest activation during activation mapping for frequent PVCs and pacing for noninducible PVCs	Not reported	Not reported	78	Unknown[a]

Included studies of ≥5 patients with available data on catheter used and acute ablation outcome.

Abbreviations: AL, anterolateral; f/u, follow-up; PL, posterolateral; PM, posteromedial; VA, ventricular arrhythmias.

[a] Because of mixed study patients with and without cardiomyopathy.

[b] Included only patients without cardiomyopathy.

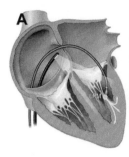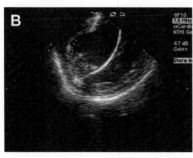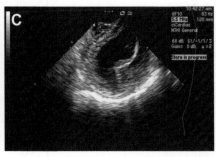

Fig. 4. (*A*) Intracardiac ultrasound is performed to assist ablation of arrhythmias rising from left anterolateral papillary muscle. (*B, C*) It allows clear visualization and confirmation of contact with the anterolateral and posteromedial muscles. ([*A*] *From* Liu XK, Barrett R, Packer DL, et al. Successful management of recurrent ventricular tachycardia by electrical isolation of anterolateral papillary muscle. Heart Rhythm 2008;5(3):481; with permission.)

other potential complications including ischemia, injury to the conduction system, and free wall rupture. The LV papillary muscles can hold firmly to the free LV wall from their base and tip (ie, tethered morphology), thus deeper ablation may theoretically cause cardiac perforation. However, some variations exist; a fingerlike morphology or more than one third of the body protruding freely in the LV cavity was reported.[34] Related to the morphologies, the fingerlike shape tends to have a long central artery branched from the nearest epicardial coronary artery that runs from the base to the tip without much anastomosis. This may be predisposed to ischemia during deep ablation, compared with the tethered morphology, which is commonly associated with a segmental branch with rich anastomosis.[34]

Efficacy of Ablation

Acute procedure success for ablation of the papillary arrhythmias (ie, elimination of targeted PVCs during the procedure) is generally fair (60%–100%).[3,8,26,35] The largest multicenter study of idiopathic ventricular arrhythmias found that ablation of the papillary arrhythmias had the lowest success rate of 60%.[3] In subjects with suspected PVC or tachycardia-induced cardiomyopathy secondary to the papillary muscle PVCs, LV ejection fraction typically normalizes. However, recurrence of similar morphology arrhythmias that require a redo ablation is common (approximately 5%–58%); subsequent procedures are often successful with an irrigated and a larger tip catheter.[4,8,26]

Predictors of successful ablation are based on limited studies. These include a smaller size of the papillary muscles assessed by CMR and the presence of Purkinje potentials at the site of ablation, which may reflect a superficial location of the arrhythmogenic substrate.[26] Clinical course during a long-term follow-up is unknown.

MALIGNANT VENTRICULAR ARRHYTHMIAS

Although papillary muscles rarely is a source of life-threatening arrhythmias, these arrhythmias may be potentially treatable by a catheter-based ablation.

Maintaining Circuits for Ventricular Fibrillation

The role of Purkinje fibers and papillary muscles in generating and maintaining VF in animal models has been suggested.[36–39] The Purkinje-ventricular muscle is a known site for a "low safety factor."[37,40,41] This condition predisposes a unidirectional block, which can lead to anchored regions of reentry. This hypothesis is based on the explanation called "source-sink mismatch." The wave front of an action potential that propagates in cardiac tissue acts as a source of the depolarizing current for the adjacent tissue (sink). The source current density must be sufficient to bring the sink to its activation threshold. If the mismatch is too large, propagation fails (source-sink mismatch), leading to the low safety factor.

In a study using a rabbit model, ablation of the papillary muscle terminated inducible VF.[42] In a porcine model, Valderrabano and colleagues[43] found that 59% of the reentrant circuits responsible for maintaining VF occurred in RV and LV papillary muscles. Subsequent histologic examination confirmed an abrupt change of the muscular fiber orientation in the region of the papillary muscles. Kim and colleagues[37] demonstrated that 78% of reentrant wave fronts involved in VF anchored to the papillary muscles and that reduction of the swine's papillary muscles resulted in the suppression of VF, supporting the source-sink mismatch hypothesis. However, it is noteworthy that studies in ischemia-associated VF offer conflicting observations. Although the LV papillary muscles were identified as areas harboring reentrant foci for type II VF (late and slow VF) in porcine and canine models, wide ablation of the papillary muscle guided by the presence of Purkinje fiber potentials only reduced the inducibility of VF in canines.[38] This may be because swine Purkinje fibers are found in the endocardium and epicardium, whereas in canine (and humans), Purkinje fibers tend to occur more endocardially.

Ventricular Fibrillation Triggered by Papillary Premature Ventricular Contractions

In humans, Haissaguerre and colleagues[44] first reported successful catheter-based ablation of idiopathic VF by targeting the Purkinje potentials. Because exits of the distal Purkinje network may be found near the papillary muscles, electrophysiologic relevance to their close approximation for the purposes of ablation has been proposed.[38] Santoro and colleagues[35] systematically reported five cases of VF/polymorphic VT triggered by papillary PVCs in structurally normal hearts. These patients tended to have a higher baseline PVC burden (mean, 19,241 beats per 24 hours) and ablation of these papillary PVCs resulted in freedom from any VF/polymorphic VT over 5 years of follow-up.

Malignant Mitral Valve Prolapse Syndrome

A subset of patients with MVP may be vulnerable to sudden cardiac death (SCD) with an annual incidence of 0.2% to 0.4%.[45,46] Recently, Basso and colleagues[19] reported 7% of young SCD victims had MVP as the only identifiable abnormality on careful clinical evaluation and autopsy. Furthermore, Sriram and colleagues[15] observed 42% of survivors from out-of-hospital arrest shared a common clinical characteristic of bileaflet MVP. These data now make it difficult to universally reassure patients with MVP.

The underlying mechanism of SCD in MVP may be involved in the mechanical effect of the redundant mitral apparatus on papillary muscles, LV outflow tract (aortomitral continuity), and the underlying Purkinje system.[15,20,47–51] This substrate formation is correlated with the presence of LGE by CMR shown in previous studies of patients with MVP with frequent PVC/nonsustained VT/aborted SCD,[19,20] and a pathologic evidence of fibrosis recently described in the Basso study.[19]

Because MVP is common with its prevalence of 2% to 3% in the general population and SCD is rare, it seems likely that MVP may pose a powerful risk factor of SCD.[46] Risk stratification, however, remains a clinical dilemma because of lacking data from prospective studies, an undiscovered

mechanistic association, and discerning the cause and effect. Emerging clinical features in particular bileaflet MVP in young adult women was thought to be a strong risk factor and was proposed for bileaflet MVP syndrome.[15,19] However, a large retrospective study of almost 6,000 cases with bileaflet MVP could not confirm this association with mortality.[46] Other proposed characteristics that have not been validated include fibrosis or scar evident on the CMR,[19,20] frequent and alternating ventricular ectopy from the papillary muscles and outflow tract regions,[15] female gender,[15,19] and repolarization (ie, T wave) abnormalities.[15,19]

SUMMARY

Ventricular arrhythmias originating from papillary muscles in a normally structural heart are not uncommon. Despite their generally benign prognosis, catheter ablation may be required for symptomatic patients or those with PVC or tachycardia-induced cardiomyopathy. Notably, ablation of papillary arrhythmias has a variable success rate because of challenges in mapping and stabilizing of the catheter. In a rare occasion, PVC arising from the papillary muscle can trigger VF and, hypothetically, papillary-Purkinje complex may also play an important role in maintaining VF.

ACKNOWLEDGMENTS

The authors thank Dr William Schleifer for his case and video, and Erica M. Ward from the Research and Academic Support Services at Mayo Clinic and Susan E. Bisco for their efforts in preparing the article.

SUPPLEMENTARY DATA

Supplementary data related to this article can be found at http://dx.doi.org/10.1016/j.ccep.2016.04.005.

REFERENCES

1. Bogun F, Desjardins B, Crawford T, et al. Post-infarction ventricular arrhythmias originating in papillary muscles. J Am Coll Cardiol 2008;51(18):1794–802.
2. Prystowsky EN, Padanilam BJ, Joshi S, et al. Ventricular arrhythmias in the absence of structural heart disease. J Am Coll Cardiol 2012;59(20):1733–44.
3. Latchamsetty R, Yokokawa M, Morady F, et al. Multicenter outcomes for catheter ablation of idiopathic premature ventricular complexes. JACC Clin Electrophysiol 2015;1(3):116–23.
4. Yamada T, McElderry HT, Okada T, et al. Idiopathic focal ventricular arrhythmias originating from the

anterior papillary muscle in the left ventricle. J Cardiovasc Electrophysiol 2009;20(8):866–72.

5. Hai JJ, Desimone CV, Vaidya VR, et al. Endocavitary structures in the outflow tract: anatomy and electrophysiology of the conus papillary muscles. J Cardiovasc Electrophysiol 2013;25(1):94–8.

6. Aliot EM, Stevenson WG, Almendral-Garrote JM, et al. EHRA/HRS expert consensus on catheter ablation of ventricular arrhythmias. Heart Rhythm 2009; 6(6):886–933.

7. Estes EH, Dalton FM, Entman ML, et al. The anatomy and blood supply of the papillary muscles of the left ventricle. Am Heart J 1966;71(3):356–62.

8. Yamada T, Doppalapudi H, McElderry HT, et al. Electrocardiographic and electrophysiological characteristics in idiopathic ventricular arrhythmias originating from the papillary muscles in the left ventricle: relevance for catheter ablation. Circ Arrhythm Electrophysiol 2010;3(4):324–31.

9. Crawford T, Mueller G, Good E, et al. Ventricular arrhythmias originating from papillary muscles in the right ventricle. Heart Rhythm 2010;7(6): 725–30.

10. Good E, Desjardins B, Jongnarangsin K, et al. Ventricular arrhythmias originating from a papillary muscle in patients without prior infarction: a comparison with fascicular arrhythmias. Heart Rhythm 2008; 5(11):1530–7.

11. Demoulin JC, Kulbertus HE. Left hemiblocks revisited from the histopathological viewpoint. Am Heart J 1973;86(5):712–3.

12. Kulbertus HE. Concept of left hemiblocks revisited. A histopathological and experimental study. Adv Cardiol 1975;14:126–35.

13. Sinnatamby CS. Last's anatomy: regional and applied. Edinburgh: Elsevier Health Sciences; 2011.

14. Yen Ho S, Ernst S. Anatomy for cardiac electrophysiologists: a practical handbook. Minneapolis (MN): Cardiotext Publishing; 2012.

15. Sriram CS, Syed FF, Ferguson ME, et al. Malignant bileaflet mitral valve prolapse syndrome in patients with otherwise idiopathic out-of-hospital cardiac arrest. J Am Coll Cardiol 2013;62(3):222–30.

16. Doppalapudi H, Yamada T, McElderry HT, et al. Ventricular tachycardia originating from the posterior papillary muscle in the left ventricle: a distinct clinical syndrome. Circ Arrhythm Electrophysiol 2008; 1(1):23–9.

17. Al'Aref SJ, Ip JE, Markowitz SM, et al. Differentiation of papillary muscle from fascicular and mitral annular ventricular arrhythmias in patients with and without structural heart disease. Circ Arrhythm Electrophysiol 2015;8(3):616–24.

18. Park K-M, Kim Y-H, Marchlinski FE. Using the surface electrocardiogram to localize the origin of idiopathic ventricular tachycardia. Pacing Clin Electrophysiol 2012;35(12):1516–27.

19. Basso C, Perazzolo Marra M, Rizzo S, et al. Arrhythmic mitral valve prolapse and sudden cardiac death clinical perspective. Circulation 2015;132(7):556–66.

20. Han Y, Peters DC, Salton CJ, et al. Cardiovascular magnetic resonance characterization of mitral valve prolapse. JACC Cardiovasc Imaging 2008;1(3): 294–303.

21. Madhavan M, Asirvatham SJ. The fourth dimension: endocavitary ventricular tachycardia. Circ Arrhythm Electrophysiol 2010;3(4):302–4.

22. Nakagawa H, Beckman KJ, McClelland JH, et al. Radiofrequency catheter ablation of idiopathic left ventricular tachycardia guided by a Purkinje potential. Circulation 1993;88(6):2607–17.

23. Nogami A. Purkinje-related arrhythmias part I: monomorphic ventricular tachycardias. Pacing Clin Electrophysiol 2011;34(5):624–50.

24. Cha YM, Lee GK, Klarich KW, et al. Premature ventricular contraction-induced cardiomyopathy: a treatable condition. Circ Arrhythm Electrophysiol 2012;5(1):229–36.

25. Usyk TP, McCulloch AD. Relationship between regional shortening and asynchronous electrical activation in a three-dimensional model of ventricular electromechanics. J Cardiovasc Electrophysiol 2003;14(Suppl 10):S196–202.

26. Yokokawa M, Good E, Desjardins B, et al. Predictors of successful catheter ablation of ventricular arrhythmias arising from the papillary muscles. Heart Rhythm 2010;7(11):1654–9.

27. Jesel L, Sacher F, Komatsu Y, et al. Characterization of contact force during endocardial and epicardial ventricular mapping. Circ Arrhythm Electrophysiol 2014;7(6):1168–73.

28. Tilz RR, Makimoto H, Lin T, et al. In vivo left-ventricular contact force analysis: comparison of antegrade transseptal with retrograde transaortic mapping strategies and correlation of impedance and electrical amplitude with contact force. Europace 2014;16(9):1387–95.

29. Abouezzeddine O, Suleiman M, Buescher T, et al. Relevance of endocavitary structures in ablation procedures for ventricular tachycardia. J Cardiovasc Electrophysiol 2010;21(3):245–54.

30. Liu X-K, Barrett R, Packer DL, et al. Successful management of recurrent ventricular tachycardia by electrical isolation of anterolateral papillary muscle. Heart Rhythm 2008;5(3):479–82.

31. Yamada T, McElderry HT, Doppalapudi H, et al. Real-time integration of intracardiac echocardiography and electroanatomic mapping in PVCs arising from the LV anterior papillary muscle. Pacing Clin Electrophysiol 2009;32(9):1240–3.

32. Yamada T, McElderry HT, Doppalapudi H, et al. Idiopathic ventricular arrhythmias originating from the left ventricular summit: anatomic concepts

relevant to ablation. Circ Arrhythm Electrophysiol 2010;3(6):616–23.

33. Roberts WC, Cohen LS. Left ventricular papillary muscles: description of the normal and a survey of conditions causing them to be abnormal. Circulation 1972;46(1):138–54.

34. Ranganathan N, Burch GE. Gross morphology and arterial supply of the papillary muscles of the left ventricle of man. Am Heart J 1969;77(4):506–16.

35. Santoro F, Biase LD, Hranitzky P, et al. Ventricular fibrillation triggered by PVCs from papillary muscles: clinical features and ablation. J Cardiovasc Electrophysiol 2014;25(11):1158–64.

36. Gornick CC, Tobler HG, Pritzker MC, et al. Electrophysiologic effects of papillary muscle traction in the intact heart. Circulation 1986;73(5):1013–21.

37. Kim YH, Xie F, Yashima M, et al. Role of papillary muscle in the generation and maintenance of reentry during ventricular tachycardia and fibrillation in isolated swine right ventricle. Circulation 1999; 100(13):1450–9.

38. Pak H-N, Kim Y-H, Lim HE, et al. Role of the posterior papillary muscle and Purkinje potentials in the mechanism of ventricular fibrillation in open chest dogs and swine: effects of catheter ablation. J Cardiovasc Electrophysiol 2006;17(7):777–83.

39. Van Herendael H, Zado ES, Haqqani H, et al. Catheter ablation of ventricular fibrillation: importance of left ventricular outflow tract and papillary muscle triggers. Heart Rhythm 2014;11(4):566–73.

40. Joyner RW, Overholt ED, Ramza B, et al. Propagation through electrically coupled cells: two inhomogeneously coupled cardiac tissue layers. Am J Physiol Heart Circ Physiol 1984;247(4):H596–609.

41. Overholt ED, Joyner RW, Veenstra RD, et al. Unidirectional block between Purkinje and ventricular layers of papillary muscles. Am J Physiol Heart Circ Physiol 1984;247(4):H584–95.

42. Pak H-N, Oh Y-S, Liu Y-B, et al. Catheter ablation of ventricular fibrillation in rabbit ventricles treated with β-blockers. Circulation 2003;108(25):3149–56.

43. Valderrábano M, Lee M-H, Ohara T, et al. Dynamics of intramural and transmural reentry during ventricular fibrillation in isolated swine ventricles. Circ Res 2001;88(8):839–48.

44. Haïssaguerre M, Shah DC, Jaïs P, et al. Role of Purkinje conducting system in triggering of idiopathic ventricular fibrillation. Lancet 2002; 359(9307):677–8.

45. Nishimura RA, McGoon MD, Shub C, et al. Echocardiographically documented mitral-valve prolapse: long-term follow-up of 237 patients. N Engl J Med 1985;313(21):1305–9.

46. Nordhues BD, Siontis KC, Scott CG, et al. Bileaflet mitral valve prolapse and risk of ventricular dysrhythmias and death. J Cardiovasc Electrophysiol 2016;27(4):463–8.

47. Akcay M, Yuce M, Pala S, et al. Anterior mitral valve length is associated with ventricular tachycardia in patients with classical mitral valve prolapse. Pacing Clin Electrophysiol 2010;33(10):1224–30.

48. Chesler E, King RA, Edwards JE. The myxomatous mitral valve and sudden death. Circulation 1983; 67(3):632–9.

49. Noseworthy PA, Asirvatham SJ. The knot that binds mitral valve prolapse and sudden cardiac death. Circulation 2015;132(7):551–2.

50. Sanfilippo AJ, Abdollah H, Burggraf GW. Quantitation and significance of systolic mitral leaflet displacement in mitral valve prolapse. Am J Cardiol 1989;64(19):1349–55.

51. Steven D, Roberts-Thomson KC, Seiler J, et al. Ventricular tachycardia arising from the aortomitral continuity in structural heart disease: characteristics and therapeutic considerations for an anatomically challenging area of origin. Circ Arrhythm Electrophysiol 2009;2(6):660–6.

Spectrum of Fascicular Arrhythmias

Raphael Sung, MD[a], Melvin Scheinman, MD[b],*

KEYWORDS

- Fascicular arrhythmia • Ventricular tachycardia • Idiopathic left ventricular tachycardia
- Intrafascicular ventricular tachycardia • Interfascicular ventricular tachycardia

KEY POINTS

- Ventricular arrhythmias originating in the ventricles include intrafascicular reentrant arrhythmias, interfascicular reentrant arrhythmias, and focal mechanism.
- Each mechanism of arrhythmia requires a unique approach for successful ablation.
- Recognition of the complex, macroscopic structure of the specialized His-Purkinje conduction system, combined with clear understanding of the electrophysiologic principles of normal and abnormal fascicular tissue properties, will help guide even the most complex arrhythmia ablations.

INTRODUCTION

Fascicular arrhythmias encompass a wide spectrum of ventricular arrhythmias that depend on the specialized conduction system, including the His, right and left bundles, left-sided fascicular bundles, and the extensive Purkinje network of fibers extending out from the fascicular bundles. These fascicular or Purkinje-dependent arrhythmias are seen in idiopathic or apparently structurally normal hearts as well as in patients after infarction and hearts with advanced conduction system disease. The mechanisms of arrhythmias are varied and include intrafascicular reentry, interfascicular reentry, and abnormal automaticity or triggered activity. Although fascicular arrhythmias in structurally normal hearts most commonly involve intrafascicular reentry, our evolving understanding of this complex entity now delineates interfascicular reentry and triggered activity or automaticity as additional mechanisms with important implications for successful ablation.

Historical Background

The original description of the conduction system and its function was described by Sunao Tawara in his monograph published in 1906. Although Purkinje first described the gelatinous network of the specialized conduction fibers, Tawara accurately demonstrated the major branch points of the His Purkinje system (HPS) and correctly addressed their role in conduction of electrical signals.[1]

Detailed anatomic and histopathologic studies of the specialized conduction system have delineated the presence of 3 main fascicles arising from the main left bundle branch (LBB).[2–4] In addition to the commonly recognized left anterior fascicle (LAF) and left posterior fascicle (LPF), a mid or upper left septal fascicle (LSF) has been well characterized anatomically, with a growing body of evidence on the electrocardiographic data supporting its role in left ventricular (LV) conduction.[5–7] The middle or septal fascicle was initial recognized by Tawara's macroscopic depiction of a trifascicular branch extending out

No conflict of interest.
[a] Community Hospital of the Monterey Peninsula, Monterey, CA, USA; [b] University of California San Francisco, 350 Parnassus Avenue, #300, San Francisco, CA 94117, USA
* Corresponding author.
E-mail address: melvin.scheinman@ucsf.edu

cardiacEP.theclinics.com

from the LBB in humans' heart,[8] with further refinement of the LSF anatomy based on reconstructed histologic transverse sections of the LBB by Demoulin and Kulbertus.[2] Their diagrammatic illustrations of the left-sided conduction system bundles in 20 normal hearts yielded the following findings (**Fig. 1**):

- Five out of 20 cases have a distinct septal fascicle extending directly from the main left bundle located between the angle formed by the LAF and LPF (cases 1, 2, 3, 4, and 14).
- Three extend directly from the proximal LAF (cases 5, 6, and 7).
- Six extend from the LPF (cases 8–13).
- Six result from the contribution of both LAF and LPF (cases 15–20).

The trifascicular nature of the LV conduction system is more clearly understood and gaining acceptance. High-density activation mapping has consistently demonstrated that there are 3 endocardial areas that are simultaneously activated, 2 representing LAF and LPF conduction, and a third area activated along the LV septum along the basal third of the midseptum.[9,10] The electrocardiogram (ECG) pattern of LSF block is more subtle than the LAF and LPF blocks. The typical ECG pattern of the LSF block includes predominant anterior forces characterized by prominent R waves particularly in leads V1 and V2, mild increase in QRS duration (typically 100–115 ms), and loss of initial septal forces characterized by loss of q wave in lead I and the left precordial leads[5,7] (**Fig. 2**). One challenge to clearer understanding of the electrical properties of the LSF may be due to significant anatomic variation resulting in divergence in its ECG characteristics across individuals. Regardless, appreciation for the distinct electrical properties of the LSF is vital to understanding and successfully managing patients with fascicular arrhythmias.

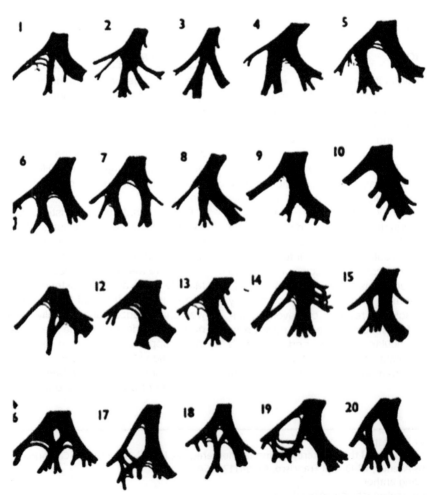

Fig. 1. The left-sided conduction system as observed in 20 normal hearts. (*From* Demoulin JC, Kulbertus HE. Histopathological examination of concept of left hemiblock. Br Heart J 1972;34:807–4; with permission.)

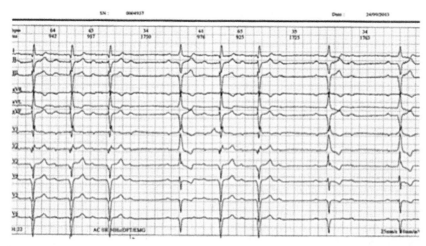

Fig. 2. A 12-lead ECG depicting second-degree atrioventricular block, underlying left anterior fascicular block, and phase 4 (bradycardia dependent) left septal fascicular block on QRS No. 4, 7, and 8. (*From* Ibarrola M, Chiale PA, Perez-Riera AR, et al. Phase 4 left septal fascicular block. Heart Rhythm 2014;11:1655–7; with permission.)

Mechanisms of Fascicular Arrhythmias

Fascicular arrhythmias occurring in apparently normal hearts include the full spectrum of ventricular arrhythmias. These arrhythmias include premature ventricular contractions (PVCs), monomorphic ventricular tachycardia (MVT), polymorphic ventricular tachycardia (PMVT), and ventricular fibrillation (VF).

There are 3 main mechanisms responsible for fascicular arrhythmias in structurally normal hearts and include the following:

1. Intrafascicular reentry (verapamil sensitive)
2. Interfascicular reentry (rare)
3. Focal (triggered and enhanced automaticity)

Fascicular ventricular tachycardia (FVT) accounts for 10% to 20% of idiopathic ventricular tachycardia (VT) cases evaluated at major electrophysiology centers.[11,12] The relative frequency of these 3 distinct mechanisms is difficult to assess given the relatively rare occurrence of some mechanisms and lack of systematic evaluation of underlying mechanism or demographics. However, based on available data, interfascicular reentry likely accounts for more than 95% of FVT, with interfascicular and focal mechanisms accounting for less than 1% to 2% each.[11–15]

Clinical Presentation of Fascicular Arrhythmias

Patients with FVT are typically younger than patients with VT with structural heart disease. Most patients are between 15 and 40 years of age, with an earlier age presentation in women, although most of the patients are male (60%–70%).[13,16–21] Common symptoms include palpitations, fatigue, dyspnea at rest and with exertion, dizziness, and presyncope.

Syncope and sudden death are rare, particularly when the mechanism involves intrafascicular reentry,[18] although focal fascicular triggers are implicated as triggers in rare cases of idiopathic PVT and ventricular fibrillation.[22] Most episodes of FVT seem to occur at rest, but episodes may also be triggered by exercise and with emotional stress.[13,23] Cases of incessant tachycardia leading to tachycardia-mediated cardiomyopathy have also been described.[21]

Intrafascicular Reentry

Intrafascicular reentrant VT is synonymous with idiopathic LV tachycardia, Belhassen VT, or verapamil-sensitive VT. Although this entity was described as early as 1972,[24] Zipes and colleagues[25] described 3 cases whereby VT was induced by atrial stimulation. All 3 patients were young (aged 14–22 years) without evidence of heart disease, and all exhibited VT morphology with right bundle branch block (RBBB) and left axis deviation (LAD) morphology. Since then, our understanding of this interesting form of tachycardia has been steadily advanced:

- There is insensitivity to multiple antiarrhythmics, including adenosine, lidocaine, ajmaline, and quinidine.[25]
- Responsiveness to verapamil: slow intravenous infusion slows tachycardia, and rapid intravenous (IV) bolus often results in VT termination.[16,25]
- There is different VT morphology with RBBB, and right axis deviation (RAD) QRS is

described with similar electrophysiologic mechanisms.[26]

- Entrainment criteria show mechanism of reentry with direct effect of verapamil on zone of slow conduction.[27]
- Ablation target of sites exhibiting late diastolic potentials or Purkinje potentials results in successful ablation.[14,28] These sites are remote from earliest ventricular activation.
- The reentrant mechanism likely involves abnormal Purkinje tissue with decremental properties, exhibiting verapamil sensitivity as well as normal Purkinje/fascicular system.[29,30]

This complex VT entity may be viewed as a simple circuit within the Purkinje network consisting of 2 limbs: antegrade and retrograde. Typically, the antegrade limb (often designated as the abnormal tissue) provides the mechanistic zone of slow conduction and is responsible for verapamil sensitivity of this tachycardia. The retrograde limb (designated as the normal fascicular tissue) provides the retrograde limb of the circuit. **Table 1** summarizes the various classification and nomenclature used in published literature of the circuit limbs responsible for intrafascicular reentry.

Nogami and colleagues[29] were the first to use an octapolar electrode catheter to characterize these potentials during both VT and sinus rhythm (SR). **Fig. 3**, from their study, demonstrates signals from a linear octapolar catheter placed along the interventricular septum within the LV as well as His bundle (His), right ventricular (RV), and select surface ECG signals. **Fig. 3**A shows antegrade activation of diastolic Purkinje potentials (P1) (LV7-8 is proximal septum, LV1-2 is more distal septum), with earliest P1 signal preceding QRS by 84 ms. Presystolic Purkinje potentials (P2) demonstrate retrograde activation during VT, with the earliest signal observed in LV1-2 with a short pre-QRS interval. **Fig. 3**B shows activation of signals during SR. P2 activation is now antegrade with increased separation from local ventricular signals as well as longer pre-QRS intervals as compared during VT.

The mechanism of intrafascicular VT is depicted by Nogami and colleagues[29] and is shown in **Fig. 4**:

- **Fig. 4**A: P1 represents abnormal Purkinje tissue exhibiting slow conduction. P2 represents normal LAF or LPF. Normal SR propagation along P2 is antegrade and exits fascicular tissue to activate myocardium. P1 activation is both antegrade in the proximal segment and retrograde in the distal segment, with collision of wavefronts in the middle.
- **Fig. 4**B: This image is the proposed circuit during VT. Initiation likely results from antegrade block along P2, but slowed antegrade conduction along P1 persists and initiates reentry with P2 participating in retrograde conduction of the VT circuit.

Although this represented paradigm is simple to understand, it is unlikely to be an exhaustive explanation for the full spectrum of intrafascicular or verapamil-sensitive forms of fascicular arrhythmias. Cases of verapamil-sensitive RBBB superior axis VT have been described that reveal the critical limb to be the LV myocardium, sometimes without participation of the LPF in the tachycardia circuit.[30,31] Furthermore, there are descriptions of retrograde conduction over the abnormal Purkinje tissue as well as LPF during VT,[30] contradicting the previously established pattern of antegrade conduction along abnormal Purkinje fibers and retrograde conduction along the LPF.[14] These differences likely represent the complexity of this multifaceted disorder, in line with the elaborate structural network of the left-sided conduction system network.

Table 1		
Classification and nomenclature of idiopathic, intrafascicular ventricular tachycardia		
Directionality of Circuit Limb	**Retrograde**	**Antegrade**
Normal vs abnormal tissue	Normal (typically left posterior fascicle or left anterior fascicle)	Abnormal (slowly conducting Purkinje fibers)
Electrogram signal nomenclature/classification	Purkinje potential P2 Fascicular potential P2	Diastolic potential Late diastolic potential Retrograde Purkinje activation P1
Location during VT	Early presystolic period (~13 ms pre-QRS)	Mid to late diastolic period (~60 ms pre-QRS)

Abbreviations: P1, diastolic Purkinje potential; P2, presystolic Purkinje potential.

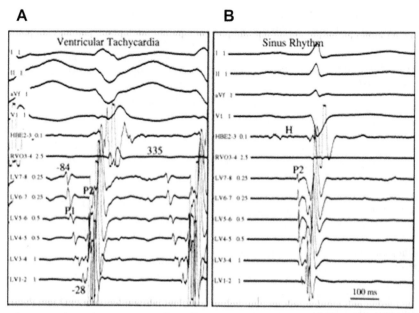

Fig. 3. Intracardiac recordings from octapolar electrode catheter. (*A*) During VT a diastolic potential (P1) and a presystolic Purkinje potential (P2) were recorded. P1 signals were activated proximal (basal) to distal (apical), with P2 signals activated distal to proximal. (*B*) During SR, recording at the same site shows only P2 signals recorded before onset of QRS. P1 signals likely represent abnormal Purkinje tissue. P2 signals likely represent signals from left posterior fascicle. H, His. (*From* Nogami A, Naito S, Tada H, et al. Demonstration of diastolic and presystolic Purkinje potentials as critical potentials in a macroreentry circuit of verapamil-sensitive idiopathic left ventricular tachycardia. J Am Coll Cardiol 2000;36:811–23; with permission.)

Initial studies implicated a fibromuscular band or false tendon as a possible anatomic substrate for FVT given their relatively high incidence in patients with idiopathic left VT (ILVT)[32] as well as elimination of VT with surgical resection of the false tendon[33] or with radiofrequency ablation.[34]

However, a study by Lin and colleagues[35] showed a high prevalence of this muscular band in 35 out of 40 consecutive patients presenting with paroxysmal supraventricular tachycardia, not statistically different from the group of patients presenting with IL VT [35] Given these data, it is

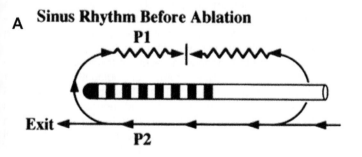

Fig. 4. The mechanism of left posterior fascicular VT. See text for details. P1, abnormal Purkinje fiber; P2, left posterior fascicle. (*Adapted from* Nogami A, Naito S, Tada H, et al. Demonstration of diastolic and presystolic Purkinje potentials as critical potentials in a macroreentry circuit of verapamil-sensitive idiopathic left ventricular tachycardia. J Am Coll Cardiol 2000;36:811–23; with permission.)

less likely that these muscular bands or false tendon play a critical role in most cases of ILVT.

Ablation of Intrafascicular Reentrant Ventricular Tachycardia

Multiple ablation approaches have been successfully described, each varying in technique. **Table 2** highlights specific characteristics/targets resulting in successful ablation in previously published studies.[12–14,23,28–30] Overall, long-term success after catheter ablation is more than 95%,[12–14,23,28–30] with rare complications that include transient LBB block,[28] left posterior fascicular block,[12] and mild increase in aortic valve regurgitation from retrograde approach.[36] Heart block was not observed following ablation of intrafascicular reentrant VT in any of the aforementioned studies.[12–14,23,28–30,36]

When targeting RBBB, LAD morphology intrafascicular VT, successful ablation locations vary extensively ranging from basal LV septum just below the LBB and extending to the apical posterior septum. Electrogram characteristics guiding successful ablation sites are also varied, ranging from targeting the earliest VT activation site to targeting the earliest Purkinje potential site as well as sites with presence of any diastolic potential.

In cases whereby VT is not inducible, but intrafascicular reentrant VT is suspected based on ECG morphology of VT, verapamil sensitivity, and pace map data during EP study, empirical ablation of VT is feasible with good long-term success. Ouyang and colleagues[30] demonstrated that retrograde Purkinje potentials (retroPP) during SR are present only in patients with documented ILVT and conspicuously absent in patients without ILVT. The earliest retroPP was targeted for ablation until no longer observed. A second ablation strategy in noninducible VT is to perform an ablation line transecting the LPF signals along the mid to distal portion of the inferior septum, extending from mid septum to the junction between septum and posterior wall. Although this was performed only in patients with documented ILVT with RBBB, LAD VT, one may hypothesize that an analogous approach may be performed for the LAF in patients with documented RBBB, RAD VT.

Although the optimal ablation strategy will vary from patient to patient, a few key points are worth remembering:

1. Successful LV ablation sites extend from base of the LV septum to the apex, and there is likely more than one successful ablation site in many cases.
2. Successful ablation electrogram characteristics of diastolic potential, Purkinje potential,

and LV exit sites are progressively more basal to apical, respectively.
3. There seems to be higher success of ablation targeting diastolic potential versus Purkinje potential and targeting Purkinje potential versus LV exit sites.
4. Published ablations of basal targets have sometimes resulted in temporary LBBB. If ablation along the basal septum must be performed, it should be done with caution to avoid high-grade conduction system damage or complete heart block.
5. Although pace maps may help confirm fascicular mechanism of VT and guide ablation targets, a perfect pace map is not necessary to guide successful ablation. Often, an imperfect pace map match may be due to concomitant capture of local myocardium along with fascicular capture and may belie a successful ablation site.

Upper Septal–Dependent Interfascicular Reentry

VT incorporating 2 or more distinct bundle or fascicular branches to form a macroreentrant circuit has been well described in patients with acquired structural heart disease with significant conduction system abnormality.[37–42] Bundle branch reentrant VT (BBRT) is the more common form, with the right and left bundles creating the two limbs of the circuit with the interventricular septum as the connecting limb.[38,39,41,42] However, interfascicular reentry involving the LAF and LPF has also been described, resulting in VT with RBBB morphology QRS and LAD versus RAD, depending on LPF versus LAF acting as the antegrade limb, respectively.[37,40,41] Significant disease within the HPS is considered a necessary component for interfascicular reentry, allowing for enough slowing in conduction to sustain stable reentry.

LSF-dependent reentrant fascicular tachycardia is a rare form of idiopathic fascicular tachycardia.[15,43] This VT exhibits a narrow QRS (less than 100 ms) and normal or right axis morphology.[43,44] Although this special VT form has been previously grouped with the traditional intrafascicular reentrant VT as described earlier, the authors have recently elucidated a unique mechanism of this uncommon form of idiopathic VT that warrants special consideration for both electrophysiology study as well as ablation techniques in comparison with typical intrafascicular VT.[15]

There are several unique properties to this form of VT that may distinguish it from typical intrafascicular VT[15,43–45]:

1. Many cases exhibit verapamil (or diltiazem) insensitivity.

Table 2
Successful ablation location and characteristics of idiopathic, intrafascicular ventricular tachycardia from larger, published data

Authors, Year	Patients	Successful Ablation Characteristics	Location of Ablation	VT Morphology
Nakagawa et al,[23] 1993	8	• Ablation of earliest P-potential (27 ± 9 ms vs 14 ± 6 ms at unsuccessful sites)	• Mid to distal posterior septum: ~one-third from apex	• RBBB, LAD
Kottkamp et al,[13] 1995	5	• Ablation at earliest endocardial activation • Ablation at complex, fractionated, mid-diastolic potential	• Basal to midapical posterior septum near left posterior fascicle	• RBBB, LAD • RBBB, RAD
Nogami et al,[14] 1998	6	• Ablation at VT exit site successful in 3 out of 6 (fused P-potential with local ventricular signal) • Remaining patients with successful ablation at diastolic P-potential sites	• VT exit: mid to distal anterolateral LV near left anterior fascicle • Diastolic P-potential: basal to midanterior septum	• RBBB, RAD
Tsuchiya et al,[28] 1999	16	• Ablation at VT exit site (earliest ventricular activation successful in 5 patients) • Ablation at earliest P-potential successful in 2 patients • Ablation at LDP site successful in 9 patients	• VT exit site: distal posterior septum • LDP site: basal anterior septum (2 patients had transient LBBB)	• RBBB, LAD
Nogami et al,[29] 2000	20	• Ablation at sites of double potential (both P1 and P2); earliest P1 not targeted because of proximity to His/LBB • If double potential not present, ablation targeting earliest ventricular activation with fused P2	• Double potential: midseptum • Single potential: middle to inferior apical septum	• RBBB, LAD
Ouyang et al,[30] 2002	9	• Inducible VT: target ablation at sites where mechanical trauma terminates VT • Target sites of diastolic potential during VT • Noninducible VT: target ablation at earliest retrograde P-potential during SR	• Not clearly reported • Some ablation sites along mid to distal posterior septum near left posterior fascicle	• RBBB, LAD
Lin et al,[12] 2005	6	• Confirm close pace map to clinical VT • Guide ablation line along sites of P-potentials	• Perpendicular ablation line to long-axis of LV • Ablation mid to distal LV at midinferior apical septum • Ablation line from midseptum to junction of septum with inferior free wall of LV	• Clinical RBBB, LAD VT; noninducible at time of EP study

Abbreviations: EP, electrophysiology; LDP, late diastolic potential; P-potential, Purkinje potential; RBBB, right bundle branch block.

2. Activation mapping of the proximal right bundle and LPF or LAF or both show near simultaneous activation, explaining narrow QRS form with LAD, RAD, or normal axis, respectively.
3. Alternating VT morphologies may be observed spontaneously or with mechanical injury (or ablation) to one of the fascicles

4. Successful ablation is performed along the upper septum between the angle formed by the LPF and LAF.

Fig. 5 shows the proposed mechanism of VT in an unusual case of a 39-year-old man with upper septal VT. He previously underwent extensive empirical LPF ablation for RBBB, LAD VT

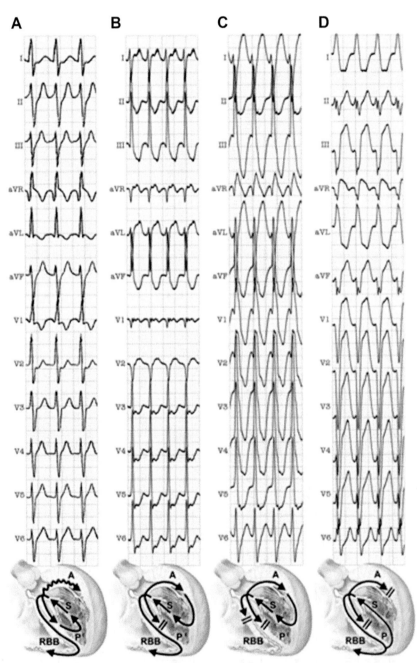

Fig. 5. VT morphologies and corresponding interfascicular circuits using upper septal fascicle. These VT morphologies were observed in the same patient following targeted ablation or mechanical injury to LPF, LAF, and right bundle branch (RBB). See text for discussion. A, left anterior fascicle; S, left septal fascicle. (*From* Sung RK, Kim AM, Tseng ZH, et al. Diagnosis and ablation of multiform fascicular tachycardia. J Cardiovasc Electrophysiol 2013;24:297–304.)

(VT1, see **Fig. 5**A), with complete left posterior fascicular block following ablation. Soon thereafter, the patient had recurrence with narrow complex RAD VT (VT2, see **Fig. 5**B). Mechanical trauma of the RBB resulted in RBBB RAD morphology VT without change in cycle length (VT3, see **Fig. 5**C), with return of narrow complex VT after several minutes.

Fig. 6 shows ECG and electrograms during narrow complex VT as depicted in **Fig. 5**B. Mapping along the proximal LAF and LPF showed antegrade conduction along both fascicles in VT and SR, with interruption of LPF signals along the basal to midseptum. Presystolic potentials (PP) were observed along the proximal to mid LAF, presumed to be LAF signals, with a PP-QRS interval of 35 ms during tachycardia. There was near-perfect pace map at this site, and concealed entrainment was confirmed with postpacing interval equal to tachycardia cycle length of 320 ms (**Fig. 7**). Tachycardia mechanism was not apparent at the time; ablation was attempted along the proximal to mid LAF, resulting in a fourth VT morphology with LBBB, LAD (VT4, see **Fig. 5**D). The authors confirmed that this fourth VT was an unusual form of BBRT, with a short HV interval during tachycardia due to zone of slow conduction along the upper septal fascicle, and parallel activation of His and RBB. Entrainment mapping confirmed that the RBB was part of the circuit,

whereas it was clearly not part of the circuit in the other VT forms. Mechanical trauma of the RBB during LBBB VT resulted in immediate termination of the BBRT with transient complete heart block, indicating antegrade block across LPF, LAF, and RBB. Fortunately, the patient recovered antegrade conduction along LAF within a few minutes.

Additional mapping along the septum adjacent to mid LAF revealed an interesting site with concealed entrainment and extremely long stimulus to QRS time, implicating capture of a fascicular potential hidden within the local myocardial signal, resulting in activation of the following (second) QRS (**Fig. 8**, see legend for more details). Mechanical trauma occurred near this site during mapping, and only nonsustained VT was inducible. Given the proximity to the LBB, no further ablation was performed; the patient remained VT free on low-dose beta-blockers for more than 4 years. **Fig. 9** shows a diagram depicting the true arrhythmia circuit responsible for this complex VT.

Following the authors' publication, a similar case was reported by Nishiuchi and colleagues[45] reporting similar findings of alternating VT morphology, unsuccessful ablation near the middle septal area where both P1 (abnormal tissue) and P2 (purported LPF) signals were visible, but successful ablation at the left upper septum where only P1, but not P2, was observed. P1-QRS and

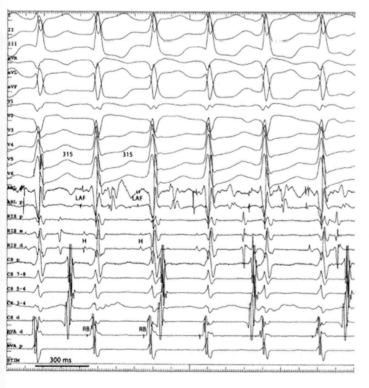

Fig. 6. ECG and electrograms of narrow complex VT, with tachycardia cycle length of 315 ms. LAF, His (H), and right bundle (RB) potentials are visualized on ablator, H, and RV catheters, respectively.

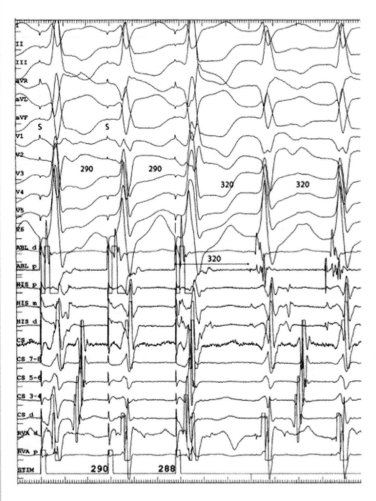

Fig. 7. ECG and electrograms during concealed entrainment from the LAF. Pacing is performed at the proximal LAF with capture of the LAF potential. Postpacing interval to the LAF is 320 ms, matching tachycardia cycle length. Stimulus to QRS interval is equal to LAF-QRS interval. Retrograde His signals are present and follow immediately after LAF activation.

P2-QRS intervals were more typical than the authors' case (57 ms and fused, respectively).

The anatomic and histopathologic studies detailed earlier support the authors' mechanistic findings that at least some of these upper septal–dependent fascicular VTs result from macroreentry involving the upper septum (typically retrograde) as the abnormal, slowly conducting, critical portion of the circuit and any combination of the LPF, LAF, and/or RBB as the antegrade limb.

Ablation of Upper Septal or Interfascicular Ventricular Tachycardia

Specific guidelines for ablation of this unique VT is challenging because of its rare occurrence. Based on the authors' experience, which is the largest to date, they recommend the following approach:

1. If possible, map and mark anatomic locations of His, RBB, LBB, LPF, and LAF during SR to help facilitate fascicular potential mapping during VT.

2. During VT, confirm reentry as mechanism by entrainment maneuvers.
3. If entrainment confirms reentry, evaluate whether conduction along proximal LAF, LPF, and RBB is antegrade or retrograde.
4. If there is no evidence of retrograde conduction along any fascicular bundle, evaluate for diastolic potentials along the upper septum in between the angle formed by the LPF and LAF.
5. Perform entrainment mapping at diastolic potential sites to confirm location is within the circuit.
6. Consider ablation at sites of diastolic potentials that are part of the VT circuit, using caution not to ablate at LBB or higher to avoid risking advanced conduction system disease or heart block.

Focal Mechanism of Fascicular Arrhythmias

Although rare, a focal mechanism (triggered or automaticity) is likely responsible for a wide spectrum of ventricular arrhythmias, including PVCs,[46] MVT,[47,48] and PVT or ventricular fibrillation.[22] The

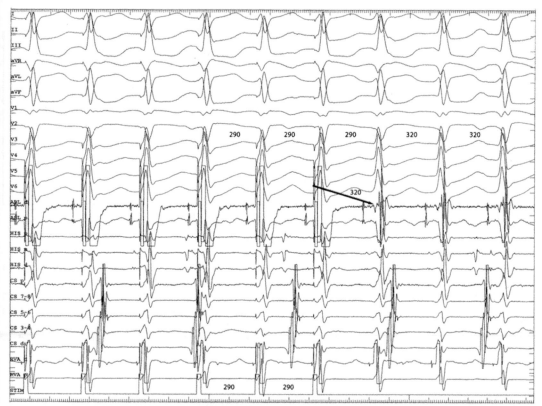

Fig. 8. Entrainment along the septal aspect of the LV near LAF. LAF Purkinje potential is seen on the ablation catheter (ABL) as a sharp, presystolic, high-frequency signal. Pacing at this site results in capture of a different fascicular potential just after start of QRS with perfect pace map. The last captured beat is the first QRS without stimulus artifact, as shown by QRS interval of 290 ms, and matches pacing interval. Postpacing interval to likely fascicular potential (fused with local ventricular signal) is equal to tachycardia cycle length, which implicates pacing site as the entrance of a very slowly conducting retrograde limb along the midseptum adjacent to LAF.

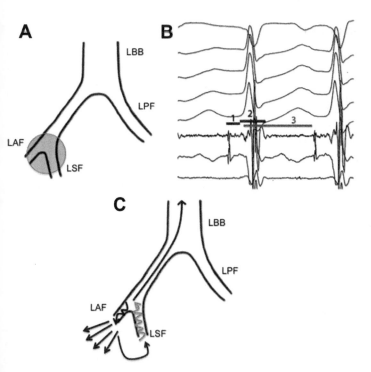

Fig. 9. VT schema. (*A*) The red highlighted area represents the local potentials being recorded from the ablation catheter, located along the midportion of the left anterior fascicle. (*B*) The blue *1* represents the timing from local left anterior fascicular capture to myocardial exit, or FP-QRS interval. The red *2* represents QRS activation time. Given the narrow QRS and right axis deviation, there is simultaneous or near-simultaneous exit from the left anterior fascicle as well as right bundle branch. The green *3* represents the very long slow conduction time along the auxiliary left septal fascicle. The left septal fascicular potential seems to precede local myocardial activation, although it starts clearly after QRS initiation. (*C*) Electrical activation sequence of the VT circuit color-coded to panel (*B*).

Table 3
Electrocardiogram characteristics distinguishing fascicular versus papillary origin of premature ventricular complex/ventricular tachycardia

Distinguishing Characteristics	Idiopathic Fascicular PVC/VT	Papillary Muscle PVC/VT
V1 pattern	rsR' (typical RBBB)	Monophasic R (atypical RBBB)
Average QRS width	127 ms	150 ms
Q wave in limb leads	Present	Typically not present
Pleomorphic ectopy	Not present	May occur
PP-QRS interval at effective site (during SR)	−29 ms	+10 ms[a]

Abbreviations: PP, Purkinje potential; PVC, premature ventricular complex; RBBB, right bundle branch block.
[a] When Purkinje potential is present.

mechanism of arrhythmia initiation, trigger, and maintenance of this diverse form of arrhythmias is not yet well understood.

Ablation of Focal Fascicular Arrhythmias

VT/PVC arising from the papillary muscle versus the left-sided fascicular system may be difficult to distinguish but may be useful for ablation planning purposes. Although overlap is present between arrhythmias arising from papillary muscle versus left-sided fascicles, **Table 3** shows some key ECG features distinguishing the two.[49]

Given the paucity of data on successful ablation approaches due to the rare occurrence of these arrhythmias, there are no well-established guidelines for safe and effective ablation. The following are suggestions/guidelines based on the authors' own unpublished experience as well as limited, published data[22,46,49]:

1. Verify that reentry is not the mechanism in cases of monomorphic fascicular VT
2. Map earliest fascicular potential during arrhythmia (PVC or monomorphic PVC). The authors think that ablation at a site proximal or distal to focus may result in persistent arrhythmia via antegrade or retrograde conduction/escape.
3. Ablations of early Purkinje potentials have been performed for successful ablation of VF originating from the fascicular system. Ablation may precipitate transient PMVT and warrant close monitoring during ablation.

SUMMARY

Mapping and ablation of the fascicular system can result in high cure rates of debilitating and potentially life-threatening arrhythmias. When approaching these arrhythmias, careful consideration of the structure of the HPS as well as their electrophysiologic properties may help guide even the most complex of arrhythmias.

The authors recommend a systematic approach to evaluation of these arrhythmias, which will guide the appropriate ablation strategy to be used, remembering that intrafascicular reentry, interfascicular reentry, and focal mechanisms vary in ablation approach.

REFERENCES

1. Suma K. Sunao Tawara: a father of modern cardiology. Pacing Clin Electrophysiol 2001;24:88–96.
2. Demoulin JC, Kulbertus HE. Histopathological examination of concept of left hemiblock. Br Heart J 1972;34:807–14.
3. Kulbertus HE. Concept of left hemiblocks revisited. A histopathological and experimental study. Adv Cardiol 1975;14:126–35.
4. Rosenbaum MB, Elizari MV. Left anterior and left posterior hemiblocks. Electrocardiographic manifestations. Postgrad Med 1973;53:61–6.
5. Ibarrola M, Chiale PA, Perez-Riera AR, et al. Phase 4 left septal fascicular block. Heart Rhythm 2014;11: 1655–7.
6. Perrin MJ, Keren A, Green MS. Electrovectorcardiographic diagnosis of left septal fascicular block. Ann Noninvasive Electrocardiol 2012;17:157–8.
7. Perez Riera AR, Ferreira C, Ferreira Filho C, et al. Electrovectorcardiographic diagnosis of left septal fascicular block: anatomic and clinical considerations. Ann Noninvasive Electrocardiol 2011;16: 196–207.
8. Elizari MV, Acunzo RS, Ferreiro M. Hemiblocks revisited. Circulation 2007;115:1154–63.
9. Durrer D, van Dam RT, Freud GE, et al. Total excitation of the isolated human heart. Circulation 1970;41: 899–912.
10. Alboni P, Malacarne C, Baggioni G, et al. Left bifascicular block with normally conducting middle fascicle. J Electrocardiol 1977;10:401–4.

11. Lerman BB, Stein KM, Markowitz SM. Mechanisms of idiopathic left ventricular tachycardia. J Cardiovasc Electrophysiol 1997;8:571–83.

12. Lin D, Hsia HH, Gerstenfeld EP, et al. Idiopathic fascicular left ventricular tachycardia: linear ablation lesion strategy for noninducible or nonsustained tachycardia. Heart Rhythm 2005;2:934–9.

13. Kottkamp H, Chen X, Hindricks G, et al. Idiopathic left ventricular tachycardia: new insights into electrophysiological characteristics and radiofrequency catheter ablation. Pacing Clin Electrophysiol 1995; 18:1285–97.

14. Nogami A, Naito S, Tada H, et al. Verapamil-sensitive left anterior fascicular ventricular tachycardia: results of radiofrequency ablation in six patients. J Cardiovasc Electrophysiol 1998;9:1269–78.

15. Sung RK, Kim AM, Tseng ZH, et al. Diagnosis and ablation of multiform fascicular tachycardia. J Cardiovasc Electrophysiol 2013;24:297–304.

16. Klein GJ, Millman PJ, Yee R. Recurrent ventricular tachycardia responsive to verapamil. Pacing Clin Electrophysiol 1984;7:938–48.

17. Nakagawa M, Takahashi N, Nobe S, et al. Gender differences in various types of idiopathic ventricular tachycardia. J Cardiovasc Electrophysiol 2002;13: 633–8.

18. German LD, Packer DL, Bardy GH, et al. Ventricular tachycardia induced by atrial stimulation in patients without symptomatic cardiac disease. Am J Cardiol 1983;52:1202–7.

19. Lin FC, Finley CD, Rahimtoola SH, et al. Idiopathic paroxysmal ventricular tachycardia with a QRS pattern of right bundle branch block and left axis deviation: a unique clinical entity with specific properties. Am J Cardiol 1983;52:95–100.

20. Ohe T, Aihara N, Kamakura S, et al. Long-term outcome of verapamil-sensitive sustained left ventricular tachycardia in patients without structural heart disease. J Am Coll Cardiol 1995;25:54–8.

21. Ward DE, Nathan AW, Camm AJ. Fascicular tachycardia sensitive to calcium antagonists. Eur Heart J 1984;5:896–905.

22. Haissaguerre M, Shoda M, Jais P, et al. Mapping and ablation of idiopathic ventricular fibrillation. Circulation 2002;106:962–7.

23. Nakagawa H, Beckman KJ, McClelland JH, et al. Radiofrequency catheter ablation of idiopathic left ventricular tachycardia guided by a Purkinje potential. Circulation 1993;88:2607–17.

24. Cohen HC, Gozo EG Jr, Pick A. Ventricular tachycardia with narrow QRS complexes (left posterior fascicular tachycardia). Circulation 1972;45:1035–43.

25. Zipes DP, Foster PR, Troup PJ, et al. Atrial induction of ventricular tachycardia: reentry versus triggered automaticity. Am J Cardiol 1979;44:1–8.

26. Ohe T, Shimomura K, Aihara N, et al. Idiopathic sustained left ventricular tachycardia: clinical and electrophysiologic characteristics. Circulation 1988;77: 560–8.

27. Okumura K, Matsuyama K, Miyagi H, et al. Entrainment of idiopathic ventricular tachycardia of left ventricular origin with evidence for reentry with an area of slow conduction and effect of verapamil. Am J Cardiol 1988;62:727–32.

28. Tsuchiya T, Okumura K, Honda T, et al. Significance of late diastolic potential preceding Purkinje potential in verapamil-sensitive idiopathic left ventricular tachycardia. Circulation 1999;99:2408–13.

29. Nogami A, Naito S, Tada H, et al. Demonstration of diastolic and presystolic Purkinje potentials as critical potentials in a macroreentry circuit of verapamil-sensitive idiopathic left ventricular tachycardia. J Am Coll Cardiol 2000;36:811–23.

30. Ouyang F, Cappato R, Ernst S, et al. Electroanatomic substrate of idiopathic left ventricular tachycardia: unidirectional block and macroreentry within the Purkinje network. Circulation 2002;105: 462–9.

31. Morishima I, Nogami A, Tsuboi H, et al. Negative participation of the left posterior fascicle in the reentry circuit of verapamil-sensitive idiopathic left ventricular tachycardia. J Cardiovasc Electrophysiol 2012;23:556–9.

32. Thakur RK, Klein GJ, Sivaram CA, et al. Anatomic substrate for idiopathic left ventricular tachycardia. Circulation 1996;93:497–501.

33. Maruyama M, Tadera T, Miyamoto S, et al. Demonstration of the reentrant circuit of verapamil-sensitive idiopathic left ventricular tachycardia: direct evidence for macroreentry as the underlying mechanism. J Cardiovasc Electrophysiol 2001;12: 968–72.

34. Wang Q, Madhavan M, Viqar-Syed M, et al. Successful ablation of a narrow complex tachycardia arising from a left ventricular false tendon: mapping and optimizing energy delivery. Heart Rhythm 2014;11:321–4.

35. Lin FC, Wen MS, Wang CC, et al. Left ventricular fibromuscular band is not a specific substrate for idiopathic left ventricular tachycardia. Circulation 1996;93:525–8.

36. Coggins DL, Lee RJ, Sweeney J, et al. Radiofrequency catheter ablation as a cure for idiopathic tachycardia of both left and right ventricular origin. J Am Coll Cardiol 1994;23:1333–41.

37. Berger RD, Orias D, Kasper EK, et al. Catheter ablation of coexistent bundle branch and interfascicular reentrant ventricular tachycardias. J Cardiovasc Electrophysiol 1996;7:341–7.

38. Caceres J, Jazayeri M, McKinnie J, et al. Sustained bundle branch reentry as a mechanism of clinical tachycardia. Circulation 1989;79:256–70.

39. Cohen TJ, Chien WW, Lurie KG, et al. Radiofrequency catheter ablation for treatment of bundle branch reentrant ventricular tachycardia: results and long-term follow-up. J Am Coll Cardiol 1991; 18:1767–73.

40. Crijns HJ, Smeets JL, Rodriguez LM, et al. Cure of interfascicular reentrant ventricular tachycardia by ablation of the anterior fascicle of the left bundle branch. J Cardiovasc Electrophysiol 1995; 6:486–92.

41. Simons GR, Sorrentino RA, Zimerman LI, et al. Bundle branch reentry tachycardia and possible sustained interfascicular reentry tachycardia with a shared unusual induction pattern. J Cardiovasc Electrophysiol 1996;7:44–50.

42. Wang PJ, Friedman PL. "Clockwise" and "counterclockwise" bundle branch reentry as a mechanism for sustained ventricular tachycardia masquerading as supraventricular tachycardia. Pacing Clin Electrophysiol 1989;12:1426–32.

43. Shimoike E, Ueda N, Maruyama T, et al. Radiofrequency catheter ablation of upper septal idiopathic left ventricular tachycardia exhibiting left bundle branch block morphology. J Cardiovasc Electrophysiol 2000;11:203–7.

44. Abdelwahab A, Sapp JL, Gardner M, et al. A case of narrow complex tachycardia. J Cardiovasc Electrophysiol 2008;19:330–1.

45. Nishiuchi S, Nogami A, Naito S. A case with occurrence of antidromic tachycardia after ablation of idiopathic left fascicular tachycardia: mechanism of left upper septal ventricular tachycardia. J Cardiovasc Electrophysiol 2013;24:825–7.

46. Ma W, Wang X, Cingolani E, et al. Mapping and ablation of ventricular tachycardia from the left upper fascicle: how to make the most of the fascicular potential? Circ Arrhythm Electrophysiol 2013;6: e47–51.

47. Gonzalez RP, Scheinman MM, Lesh MD, et al. Clinical and electrophysiologic spectrum of fascicular tachycardias. Am Heart J 1994;128:147–56.

48. Rodriguez LM, Smeets JL, Timmermans C, et al. Radiofrequency catheter ablation of idiopathic ventricular tachycardia originating in the anterior fascicle of the left bundle branch. J Cardiovasc Electrophysiol 1996;7:1211–6.

49. Good E, Desjardins B, Jongnarangsin K, et al. Ventricular arrhythmias originating from a papillary muscle in patients without prior infarction: a comparison with fascicular arrhythmias. Heart Rhythm 2008;5: 1530–7.

Polymorphic Ventricular Tachycardia/Ventricular Fibrillation and Sudden Cardiac Death in the Normal Heart

Ashok J. Shah, MD[a],*, Meleze Hocini, MD[b], Arnaud Denis, MD[b],
Nicolas Derval, MD[b], Frederic Sacher, MD[b], Pierre Jais, MD[b],
Michel Haissaguerre, MD[b],*

KEYWORDS

- Polymorphic ventricular tachycardia • Ventricular fibrillation • Sudden cardiac death
- Electrical storm • Primary electrical disease • Normal heart • Catheter mapping • Ablation

KEY POINTS

- Polymorphic ventricular tachycardia (PMVT) and ventricular fibrillation (VF), due to primary electrical diseases or idiopathic VF, are responsible for about 10% of sudden cardiac deaths (SCDs).
- Despite multimodality secondary prevention of SCD including the avoidance of provocative agents and circumstances, up to 20% of patients experience recurrent episodes of PMVT/VF or electrical storms.
- PMVT/VF is largely triggered by premature ventricular ectopic beats (PVBs), which occur frequently in isolation around the period of electrical storm.
- In the majority of patients with primary PMVT/VF, the triggering PVBs can be mapped and localized to the peripheral Purkinje system of both ventricles.
- Right ventricular outflow tract is the most likely site of origin of culprit PVBs in Brugada syndrome.

INTRODUCTION

Polymorphic ventricular tachycardia (PMVT) and ventricular fibrillation (VF) are the most life-threatening, complex, cardiac rhythm disorders.[1] Referring to heart as normal in a patient with sudden cardiac death (SCD) sounds antithetical. However, normal conventionally refers to its structure and vascular supply examined using techniques like echocardiogram and angiogram and in the era of advanced imaging, possibly also cardiac computed tomography (CT), MRI and PET.

Although cardiac asystole has increasingly become the more common arrhythmic cause of SCD events, PMVT and VF are still associated with a substantial number of them.[2–4] About 90% of SCD events occur in a diseased heart, the most common being the coronary artery disease.[5,6] Coronary arterial abnormalities, dilated and hypertrophic cardiomyopathies, infiltrative disorders, and valvular or congenital cardiac disorder are not found in the remaining about 10% events where the heart is considered structurally normal.[6] It is rare to have spontaneous PMVT/VF in the absence of a known structural or electrical cardiac abnormality. An arrhythmic event resulting from an unknown cause is labeled as idiopathic. Primary electrical abnormalities result from mutated genes encoding proteins involved in handling ion movements in the heart.

[a] Cardio Vascular Services, South Consulting Suites, Peel Health Campus, 110 Lakes Road, Mandurah, Western Australia 6210, Australia; [b] Department of Electrophysiology and Cardiac Pacing, Hôpital Cardiologique du Haut Lévêque, Avenue de Magellan, Pessac Cedex 33604, France
* Corresponding author.
E-mail addresses: drashahep@gmail.com; michel.haissaguerre@chu-bordeaux.fr

Card Electrophysiol Clin 8 (2016) 581–591
http://dx.doi.org/10.1016/j.ccep.2016.04.007
1877-9182/16/$ – see front matter © 2016 Elsevier Inc. All rights reserved.

Because they manifest as electrocardiographic abnormalities but do not cause alterations in gross cardiac structure, the heart is regarded as normal. These disorders include long QT syndrome, Brugada syndrome, catecholaminergic polymorphic VT, short QT syndrome, and early repolarization syndrome.[7] However, Brugada syndrome is associated with epicardial late potential strongly suggestive of underlying structural changes.[8]

This article presents a clinical review of the electrophysiological management of PMVT/VF in a structurally normal heart (**Table 1**).

OVERVIEW OF MANAGEMENT

PMVT and VF are rapidly lethal arrhythmias. Implantable cardiac defibrillator (ICD) implantation is unequivocally the gold standard, first-line treatment in patients who have survived SCD (secondary prevention) and in the majority of subjects at high-risk of SCD (primary prevention).[7] ICD prolongs survival without influencing the arrhythmogenic substrate.[7] Antiarrhythmic drugs like beta-blockers, quinidine, mexilitine, and flecainide (table) complement ICDs in secondary prevention of PMVT/VF of different etiologies.[7] Drugs are also recommended as the first-line treatment for primary prevention in some forms of SCD.[7] Similarly, surgical sympathetic denervation has also been advocated and proven beneficial in secondary prevention of some cardiac electrical disorders.[7]

Despite multimodality management of SCD including the avoidance of provocative agents and circumstances, up to 20% of patients experience recurrent episodes of PMVT/VF or electrical storms. Such a situation acutely increases the mortality. In the survivors, storm deteriorates the quality of physical life and has an adverse impact psychologically from multiple device therapies delivered within a short period of time.[9] Drugs like isoproterenol, amiodarone, beta-blockers, and lidocaine have been used in life-threatening arrhythmias with variable efficacy and inconsistent benefits.

Catheter ablation of PMVT/VF has been undertaken as a life-saving measure when drugs and, fail to control incessant runs of arrhythmias. The premature ventricular beats (PVBs) triggering storm recur in isolation thereby serving as tangible targets for catheter mapping and ablation of these unmappable arrhythmias. The electrophysiological characteristics of PMVT/VF and its ectopic triggers have been described in various electrical substrates of structurally normal heart in the following sections.

MAPPING AND ABLATION OF POLYMORPHIC VENTRICULAR TACHYCARDIA/VENTRICULAR FIBRILLATION

Invasive catheter mapping of PMVT/VF targeting culprit PVBs gets facilitated and ablation yields best results when it is undertaken as close to the storm as possible. If the procedure is delayed, rarity or absence of spontaneous culprit PVCs will reduce the long-term clinical success rate of pace-map based procedure in the absence of any known and reliable provocative agent. Patients with few monomorphic PVBs have a high probability of successful ablation in contrast to those with pleomorphic PVBs arising from a wider area. In addition to being a life-saving therapy, it may provide cure at best or reduce arrhythmia burden at least, if successful.

The best approach is to ablate when the clinical PVC load is high around the time of frequent episodes of VF. Otherwise, there is no reliable method to provoke the clinical PVCs. The authors have anecdotally used atrial pacing, class I antiarrhythmic drugs, isoproterenol, Ca++, pacing induced sinus pause to provoke clinical PVC individualy, but the results are not consistent.

Frequent PMVT/VF needs to be controlled to allow mapping of clinical PVCs, requiring individually beta-blockers in catecholergic arrhythmias, verapamil in short coupled ectopies and IVF, or isoproterenol in acute storm due to abnormal early repolarization/Brugada syndrome/idiopathic VF.

Idiopathic Ventricular Fibrillation

Aizawa and colleagues[10] first reported successful suppression of electrical storms after ablation of premature ventricular beats located in the posterolateral wall of the left ventricle. Haissaguerre and colleagues[11] described ablation of

Table 1 Primary electrical diseases	
Disorder	**Drug**
Long QT syndrome	Beta blockers mexilitene in LQT3
Brugada syndrome	Quinidine
Catecholarminergic polymorphic ventricular tachycardia	Nadolol, verapmail, flecainide
Abnormal early repolarization syndrome	Quinidine
Idiopathic VF	Quinidine

idiopathic VF in 27 patients by mapping and targeting PVB with short coupling interval initiating the VF. The triggering PVBs were mapped and localized to the peripheral Purkinje system of both ventricles in 23 of 27 patients and to the right ventricular outflow tract (RVOT) myocardium in the remaining minority (**Fig. 1**).

They represent the locations of PVCs.

Purkinje arborization

The specialized His-Purkinje conduction system, comprised of approximately 1% of biventricular mass, is responsible for rapid synchronous activation of the remainder 99% of myocardial tissue.

The complex architecture of the peripheral Purkinje network and the differences in the functional properties of Purkinje cells and its contiguous myocardium provide distal Purkinje–myocardial junctional tissue with an arrhythmogenic role in PMVT/VF. Distal Purkinje fibres have been recognized as the most frequent site of VF-triggering PVB emitted during the vulnerable period of cardiac repolarization.[12–14]

Characteristics of culprit premature ventricular ectopic beats

Recording a 12-lead ECG morphology of the VF-triggering PVB is critical in localizing the precise site of origin and guides detailed intracardiac

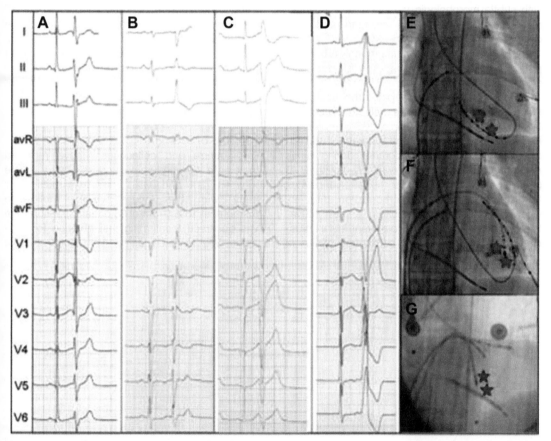

Fig. 1. Triggered VF Twelve-lead ECGs (*left*) and their corresponding location in the anteroposterior fluoroscopic view (*right, red asterisks*). The origin of ventricular premature beat (VPB) triggering VF was the left Purkinje either at the posterior (*A*) or the anterior (*B*) insertion, the right Purkinje (*C*), and the right ventricular outflow track (*D*). Related fluoroscopic views with a decapolar catheter inserted in the left ventricle (*E, F*), an ablation catheter inserted in the right ventricle (*G*), and a quadripolar catheter inserted at the His position (*E–G*). Ventricular premature beat originating in the left Purkinje system (*A, B* and related anteroposterior fluoroscopic view) produce more variable 12-lead ECG patterns, reflecting the more complex and extended Purkinje arborization on the left. VPBs originating in the right Purkinje system (*C* and related anteroposterior fluoroscopic view) typically have a left bundle-branch block pattern with left superior axis. VPBs originating from the right ventricular outflow track (*D*) have the classical aspect with a left bundle-branch block pattern and an inferior axis. (*From* Knecht S, Sacher F, Wright M, et al. Long-term follow-up of idiopathic ventricular fibrillation ablation: a multicenter study. J Am Coll Cardiol 2009;54(6):524; with permission.)

mapping of the culprit PVB. It is a routine in the authors' laboratory to continuously record 12-lead ECG at the bedside in patients who are candidates for invasive mapping and ablation of refractory PMVT/VF. The chest lead positions are marked to precisely match the morphology of PVCs on the ECG undertaken in the EP lab.

The culprit premature ventricular beats that originate from the left ventricle, are positive in V1 and produce more variable 12-lead ECG patterns, reflecting the more complex and extended Purkinje arborization on the left than the right (see **Fig. 1**A, B). They have a shorter mean QRS duration of less than 120 ms. Premature beats that originate from the right ventricle are negative in V1, with inferior or superior axis (see **Fig. 1**C, D), with subtle morphologic variations and a longer mean QRS duration (~145 ms) than beats that originate from the left ventricle.[11,14]

Left Purkinje branches are intermingly arborized, providing quicker activation than single distal arborization of RBB.

During intra-cardiac mapping, the source of PVB is localized by the earliest electrograms relative to the onset of the ectopic QRS complex. An initial sharp potential (<10 ms in duration) preceding the ventricular electrograms during sinus rhythm (<15 ms early) as well as during PVB (>15 ms early) indicates that the latter originates from the distal Purkinje arborization (**Fig. 2**), whereas its absence at the site of earliest activation indicates an origin from ventricular muscle.[11,14] Haissaguerre and colleagues observed that the conduction delay from the Purkinje network to the myocardium was variable but shorter in the right than left ventricle. Dissociated/blocked Purkinje potentials were also observed in some patients (**Fig. 3**). During couplets or triplets of PVBs, each complex was preceded by a Purkinje potential, with variable conduction time.[11,14]

The culprit PVBs have been demonstrated to originate from sites other than the cardiac conduction system (eg, the right ventricular outflow tract [RVOT][11] [see **Fig. 1**D], the left ventricular outflow tract [LVOT], and papillary muscles).[15]

In idiopathic PMVT/VF, Purkinje triggers are the primary targets for ablation. Radiofrequency current application targeting these beats usually produces a spurt of ectopics and/or PMVT/VF with subsequent gradual disappearance of the PVBs and abolition of the local Purkinje potentials. Ablation is extended about 1 to 2 cm around the arrhythmogenic site to prune the regional Purkinje arborization. After ablation, minimal/minor nonspecific QRS prolongation not fulfilling the criteria of bundle-branch block may be observed.

Outcome of ablation

Haissaguerre and colleagues[11] have reported immediate (procedural) success rates range between 73% and 88%.[14,16,17] In a multicenter study with the longest-available follow-up (63 months),18% (7 out of 38 patients), recurrence was observed, confirming that ablation for idiopathic VF, targeted at its ventricular ectopic

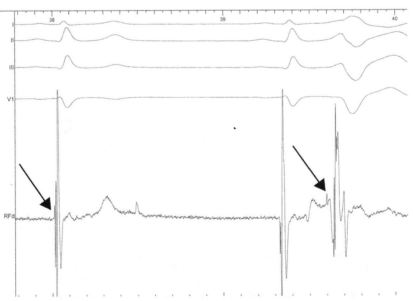

Fig. 2. Purkinje Triggered ectopy. Distal Purkinje potential is marked by black arrows in sinus rhythm. During an ectopic beat, Purkinje potential distinctly stands out preceding the local ventricular electrogram.

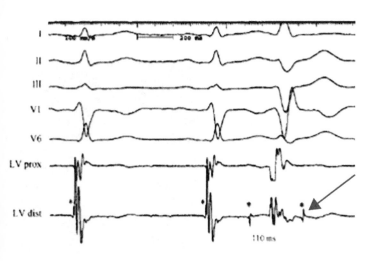

Fig. 3. Purkinje potentials (*asterisk*) precede the local ventricular ECG in sinus rhythm and ectopy. Blocked Purkinje potential is marked by a red arrow.

triggers, effectively prevents VF recurrence in the majority of this high-risk population.[16] Among 7 patients experiencing recurrence, a second procedure was successfully undertaken in five. Overall, ablation provided complete freedom from recurrent VF or substantially reduced the event rate.[16]

Van Herendael and colleagues[15] reported outcome of ablation of PMVT/VF in nonstructural heart disease targeting Purkinje and non-Purkinje sources of culprit PVBs. Acute complete success rate was reported in 89% patients. At median 418 days (IQR 144 - 866), 33% patients had recurrence. (Apologies, 67% patients had no recurrence [3 out of 9 had recurrence]).

Additionally, there are a few of individually reported cases describing success with catheter ablation of refractory PMVT/VF.[18–22]

Long QT Syndrome

With the facilitatory background of enhanced dispersion of repolarization in long-QT syndrome, the bench mechanism of torsades de pointes/VF appears to be early after depolarization (PVB) triggered nonstationary (unstable), localized reentrant arrhythmia with variable propagation in the myocardium.[23–26] In clinical practice, Purkinje fibers have also been implicated as sources of torsades-triggering PVBs.[27] Endocardial ablation suppressed spontaneous arrhythmias; however, new sources could generate arrhythmias, indicating that the Purkinje tissue was an important, but not the sole, trigger of long QT-related arrhythmias.[28]

Catheter ablation of culprit PVB triggering VF has offered arrhythmia free survival in patients with long QT syndrome refractory to conventional treatment.[29–31] Haissaguerre and colleagues[27] described mapping and ablation of PVBs-triggering arrhythmia in four patients with LQTS.

The triggering PVB was monomorphic in 2 patientsand polymorphic and repetitive (sometimes bidirectional) with a positive QRS morphology in lead V1 in the other 2. The initiating PVB arose from the distal left Purkinje fibers in 3 out of 4 patients and from the RVOT in the remaining 1 patient. The latter was repetitive, lasting 3 to 45 beats, with varying cycle lengths of 280 to 420 milliseconds. Ablation of the triggers in the distal Purkinje fibers and RVOT resulted in no recurrence during mean follow-up of 24 months.

In a case reported by Tan and colleagues,[29,30] recurrent VF was triggered by unifocal PVBs in a 16-year-old patient on maximally tolerated doses of a β-blocker. The culprit PVB was localized to the LVOT region just below the aortic valve area and was successfully ablated (**Fig. 4**). No arrhythmia recurred during the follow-up of 18 months.

Brugada Syndrome

Unlike long QT syndrome, the underlying electrophysiological mechanism of Brugada syndrome remains ambiguous. Initially proposed as an abnormality of repolarization, recent clinical studies have called it a disorder of delayed depolarization. A bench study found heterogeneity in the repolarization of the canine right ventricular myocardium as a cause of phase 2 re-entry triggered short coupled PVBs initiating VF.[23] The characteristic ECG feature of Brugada syndrome involves the junction of QRS and ST segment in addition to the ST and T components. So, the delayed depolarization of the RVOT myocardial segment could not be completely be ruled out and was hypothesized later in association with microscopic structural abnormalities in the arrhythmogenic RVOT of an explanted human heart.[31]

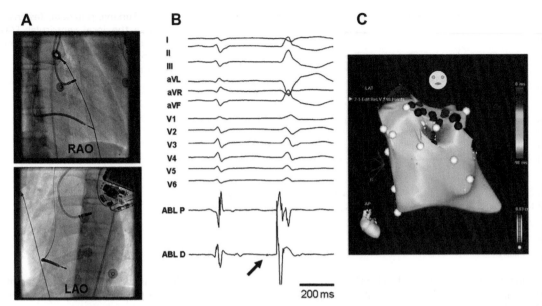

Fig. 4. Catheter ablation of the PVCs triggering recurrent VF episodes in a patient with long QT syndrome. (*A*) Fluoroscopic images (*right and left anterior oblique views*) of the ablation catheter at the site of origin of the premature ventricular complexes. (*B*) Twelve-lead surface ECG and ablation signal at earliest site (30 ms ahead of PVC onset). Note inferior axis of PVC and small Purkinje potential (PP- *thick arrow*) visible just before premature ventricular complex onset. (*C*) CARTO map of left ventricle (*anterior view*) showing multiple ablation points (*brown circles*) below the aortic valve area at the earliest site of triggering premature ventricular complexes. Coronary angiography (not shown) was performed to confirm that the ablation site was at a safe distance away from the epicardial coronary arteries. LAO, left anterior oblique view; RAO, right anterior oblique view. (*From* Tan VH, Yap J, Hsu LF, et al. Catheter ablation of ventricular fibrillation triggers and electrical storm. Europace 2012;14(12):1691; with permission.)

Clinically, PVBs triggering PMVT/VF have been mapped and ablated largely in the RVOT (see **Fig. 1**D).[27,32,33] Nademanee and colleagues[34] mapped the substrate in the RVOT instead of the PVB triggers of PMVT/VF in 9 patients with BrS and refractory arrhythmia. The substrate was characterized by abnormally low-voltage and fractionated ventricular ECGs. They were found to have prolonged duration and were markedly delayed in sinus rhythm, suggestive of slow conduction in the region. These abnormal ECGs were exclusively localized in a cluster over the epicardium of the anterior aspect of the RVOT. Catheter ablation targeting the abnormal arrhythmogenic substrate suppressed VT/VF episodes completely in 8 of 9 patients at 20 plus or minus 6 months follow-up. Interestingly, catheter ablation over the RVOT resulted in normalization of the Brugada ECG pattern in 5 of 9 patients also described (**Fig. 5**) by Shah and colleagues.[35] These findings are consistent with the delayed depolarization school of thought.

Catecholaminergic Polymorphic Ventricular Tachycardia

Catecholaminergic polymorphic VT (CPVT) is a genetic disorder of cardiac Ca^{+2} handling proteins.[36]

It affects young people who present with recurrent syncope or SCD from bidirectional VT itself or secondary to its degeneration into polymorphic VT/VF triggered by a surge in catecholamine levels due to physical or emotional outburst.[37] Pharmacologic (nadolol) and surgical sympatholysis are effective in prevention of arrhythmias.

PVBs triggering recurrent arrhythmias have been mapped and ablated successfully, albeit there is only 1 such report available in the literature.[38] The culprit PVBs originated not only from the left Purkinje system (Right bundle branch block morphology with superior axis), but also from a myocardial source (left coronary cusp) (**Fig. 6**). The multiplicity of the origin of ectopics makes ablation target sites nonspecific in CPVT.

Short QT Syndrome

Short QT syndrome is a manifestation of mutations causing hyperfunction of the delayed rectifier outward potassium current or hypofunction of the inward calcium current. These result in a shortening of the repolarization period and an increase in transmural dispersion of repolarization, which explains the main features of this syndrome: short QT interval, short atrial and ventricular effective

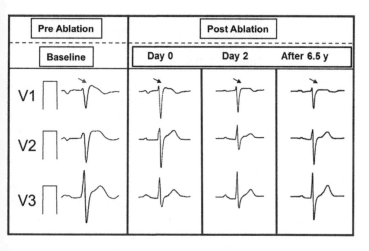

Fig. 5. Abolition of Brugada syndrome ECG by regional ablation. Arrows point to the change in the J point. (*From* Shah AJ, Hocini M, Lamaison D, et al. Regional substrate ablation abolishes Brugada syndrome. J Cardiovasc Electrophysiol 2011;22(11):1290; with permission.)

refractory periods, and, as a result of them, susceptibility to AF and VF.[39]

PMVT/VF, responsible for syncope and SCD in short QT syndrome, has no specific association with activity, rest, sleep, or noise like in other channelopathies.[39] Although ICD remains the first line of treatment in this rare electrical disease, the role of catheter mapping and ablation remains uninvestigated.

Abnormal Early Repolarization Syndrome

Abnormal early repolarization (AER) is the most recently identified primary electrical disorder of structurally normal heart. Inferolateral early repolarization was recognized as an arrhythmogenic abnormality after Haissaguerre and colleagues[17] reported significantly higher prevalence (31% vs 5%) of it in survivors of out-of-hospital SCD in comparison with healthy controls. Although the name suggests that this is a cardiac repolarization pathology, the precise mechanism is still debated. Yan and Antzelevitch proposed discrepant phase 1 of epicardial action potential relative to that of the endocardium as a cause of terminal QRS slur or notch, the J-wave.[40] Such an enhanced repolarization heterogeneity increases the susceptibility to PMVT/VF, which is triggered by phase 2

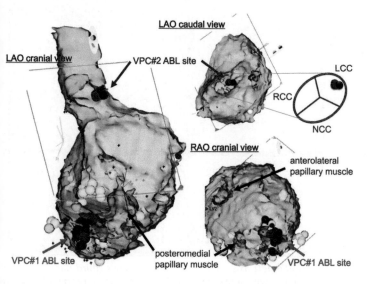

Fig. 6. Electroanatomic mapping merged with contrast-enhanced CT. Red tags indicate the ABL sites. Blue tags indicate the sites with perfect pace mapping, and yellow tags indicate the sites with Purkinje potentials during sinus rhythm. The sites with perfect pace mapping and the earliest activation for VPC #1 were localized in the inferoseptal site adjacent to the base of the posteromedial papillary muscle (*red arrow*). Successful ablation site of VPC #2 was on the left coronary cusp (*blue arrow*). ABL indicates ablation; LAO, left anterior oblique; LCC, left coronary cusp; NCC, noncoronary cusp; RAO, right anterior oblique; RCC, right coronary cusp; VPC, ventricular premature contraction. (*From* Kaneshiro T, Naruse Y, Nogami A, et al. Successful catheter ablation of bidirectional ventricular premature contractions triggering ventricular fibrillation in catecholaminergic polymorphic ventricular tachycardia with RyR2 mutation. Circ Arrhythm Electrophysiol 2012;5(1):e16; with permission.)

re-entry mediated PVB.[40] The arrhythmia is considered to be maintained by transmural reentry across the heterogeneous substrate in bench experiments.

Among 8 patients with AER and refractory electrical storm, Haissaguerre and colleagues[17] mapped 26 PVBs triggering PMVT/VF in the inferior and/or lateral left ventricular myocardium in concurrence with the ECG localization of the abnormal repolarization. There was no evidence of delayed activation of the arrhythmogenic region in the form of late or fractionated local ECG. Therefore, pathologic J-wave was not considered to have been caused by delayed depolarization, reinforcing the repolarization hypothesis. The culprit PVBs originated from the ventricular myocardium or Purkinje tissue. Catheter ablation successfully eliminated them in 5 (63%) patients and controlled the storm.

Recently, Latcu and colleagues[41] described successful ablation of the left ventricular substrate in inferior AER in a 57-year-old man with recurrent uncontrolled VF. The culprit PVBs were rare, but pace mapping confirmed their origin from the distal left posterior fascicular Purkinje network. Minimally delayed local activation was noted at this site, where catheter ablation led to elimination of ECG features of inferior AER (**Fig. 7**). At 2 months, no arrhythmia recurrence was observed.

LATEST INSIGHTS FROM NONINVASIVE MAPPING OF CLINICAL POLYMORPHIC VENTRICULAR TACHYCARDIA/VENTRICULAR FIBRILLATION

Although the understanding of VF mechanisms continues to improve, the mechanistic differences between VF depending on the causative factor remain unknown. Possibly, the ventricular substrate underlying VF is different in different pathologies.

Superficially, VF appears to be random and disorganized. However, detailed epicardial mapping suggests the coexistence of electrical rotors and disorganized activity in induced VF in patients with preserved ventricular function during open heart surgery. VF rotors have been studied in the context of ischemia and scar using animal models and explanted human hearts.[42]

The authors have performed noninvasive mapping of human VF in vivo in a broad population to characterize drivers involved in the maintenance of early phase of human VF. Mapping procedures were performed during VF using accurate biventricular geometry relative to an array of 252 body surface electrodes; VF episodes were either spontaneous or induced by programmed stimulation The reconstructed epicardial unipolar VF ECGs were acquired before defibrillation and signal processed to characterize frequency, activation, and location of focal or re-entrant drivers maintaining VF.

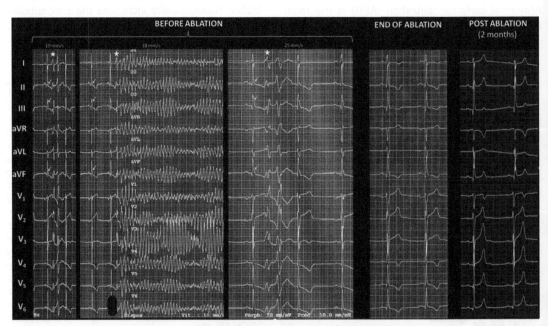

Fig. 7. Monomorphic initiating PVC (*star; right-bundle, left axis*) at 10 mm/s and 25 mm/s (*third panel*). J-wave notching was continuously present in the inferior leads, with a maximal amplitude in lead III, ranging between 3 and 3.5 mm. Right panels: ECG recordings after catheter ablation showing persistent disappearance of the J-wave notching. (*From* Latcu DG, Bun SS, Zarqane N, et al. Ablation of left ventriculsar substrate in early repolarization syndrome. J Cardiovasc Electrophysiol 2016;27(4):491; with permission.)

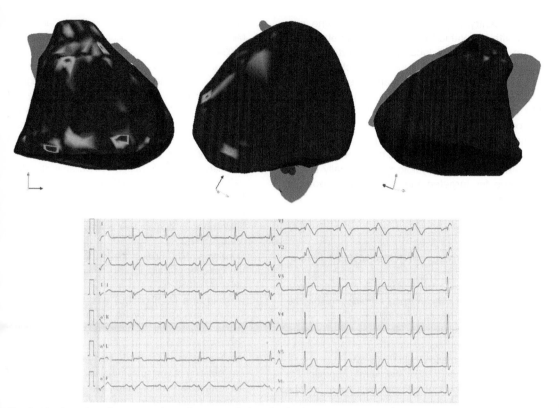

Fig. 8. Noninvasive phase mapping of VF revealed multiple driver regions involving the right ventricle in a 52-year-old male with Brugada syndrome and type I ECG pattern. (*Top*) Cluster of re-entrant drivers (*red*) involving the right ventricular outflow tract and middle and lower anterior right ventricle (RV). (*Bottom*) ECG at baseline shows Brugada pattern in V1-3.

At each instant, VF was driven by a limited number of wave fronts spanning across large surface areas that emanated from focal breakthroughs and re-entrant activity regions. Type and spatio-temporal behavior of driver activities varied considerably among individuals and underlying heart disease, ranging from discrete regions/sources responsible for the whole fibrillatory activity to mechanisms extending diffusely to both ventricles. Patients with Brugada syndrome were characterized by clustered driver domains in the right ventricle (**Fig. 8**), while idiopathic VF showed

Anterior   Inferior   Posterolateral

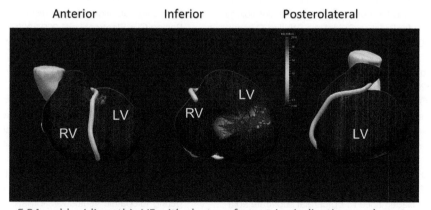

F 54 y old - Idiopathic VF with cluster of reentries indicating a substrate
target in inferior LV — ablation resulted in VF free outcome

Fig. 9. Noninvasive phase mapping of idiopathic VF revealed a cluster of re-entrant drivers in the inferior left ventricle (LV) in a 54-year-old female. RV, right ventricle.

diffuse reentry trajectories. However, some patients with idiopathic VF showed a discrete driver region, suggesting a localized substrate (**Fig. 9**) imperceptible with current imaging techniques. In a subset of patients without mappable VF triggers and frequent VF recurrences, the authors successfully ablated driver regions, resulting in VF-free outcome.

The authors strongly believe that VF mapping in vivo in such way will provide new and important insights in VF pathophysiology, potentially opening paths for targeted therapies and/or optimal defibrillation.

REFERENCES

1. Zipes D, Wellens H. Sudden cardiac death. Circulation 1998;98:2334–51.
2. Rea TD, Eisenberg MS, Sinibaldi G, et al. Incidence of EMS-treated out-of-hospital cardiac arrest in the United States. Resuscitation 2004;63:17–24.
3. Atwood C, Eisenberg MS, Herlitz J, et al. Incidence of EMS- treated out-of-hospital cardiac arrest in Europe. Resuscitation 2005;67:75–80.
4. Ewy GA, Sanders AB. Alternative approach to improving survival of patients with out-of-hospital primary cardiac arrest. J Am Coll Cardiol 2013;61:113–8.
5. Morrison LJ, Neumar RW, Zimmerman JL, et al. Strategies for improving survival after in-hospital cardiac arrest in the United States: 2013 consensus recommendations: a consensus statement from the American Heart Association. Circulation 2013;127(14):1538–63.
6. Zipes DP, Camm AJ, Borggrefe M, et al. ACC/AHA/ESC 2006 guidelines for management of patients with ventricular arrhythmias and the prevention of sudden cardiac death: a report of the American College of Cardiology/American Heart Association Task Force and the European Society of Cardiology Committee for Practice Guidelines (Writing Committee to Develop Guidelines for Management of Patients With Ventricular Arrhythmias and the Prevention of Sudden Cardiac Death). J Am Coll Cardiol 2006;48(5):e247–346.
7. Priori SG, Wilde AA, Horie M, et al. HRS/EHRA/APHRS expert consensus statement on the diagnosis and management of patients with inherited primary arrhythmia syndromes: document endorsed by HRS, EHRA, and APHRS in May 2013 and by ACCF, AHA, PACES, and AEPC in June 2013. Heart Rhythm 2013;10(12):1932–63.
8. Wilde AA, Nademanee K. Epicardial substrate ablation in Brugada syndrome: time for a randomized trial! Circ Arrhythm Electrophysiol 2015;8(6):1306–8.
9. Tomzik J, Koltermann KC, Zabel M, et al. Quality of life in patients with an implantable cardioverter defibrillator: a systematic review. Front Cardiovasc Med 2015;2. http://dx.doi.org/10.3389/fcvm.2015.00034.
10. Aizawa Y, Tamura M, Chinushi M, et al. An attempt at electrical catheter ablation of the arrhythmogenic area in idiopathic ventricular fibrillation. Am Heart J 1992;123(1):257–60. Available at: http://www.ahjonline.com/article/0002-8703(92)90786-U/abstract.
11. Haissaguerre M, Shoda M, Jais P, et al. Mapping and ablation of idiopathic ventricular fibrillation. Circulation 2002;106(8):962–7. Available at: http://circ.ahajournals.org/content/106/8/962.full.pdf.
12. Hooks DA, Berte B, Yamashita S, et al. New strategies for ventricular tachycardia and ventricular fibrillation ablation. Expert Rev Cardiovasc Ther 2015;13(3):263–76.
13. Scheinman MM. Role of the His-Purkinje system in the genesis of cardiac arrhythmia. Heart Rhythm 2009;6(7):1050–8.
14. Haissaguerre M, Shah DC, Jais P, et al. Role of Purkinje conducting system in triggering of idiopathic ventricular fibrillation. Lancet 2002;359(9307):677–8.
15. Van Herendael H, Zado ES, Haqqani H, et al. Catheter ablation of ventricular fibrillation: importance of left ventricular outflow tract and papillary muscle triggers. Heart Rhythm 2014;11(4):566–73.
16. Knecht S, Sacher F, Wright M, et al. Long-term follow-up of idiopathic ventricular fibrillation ablation: a multicenter study. J Am Coll Cardiol 2009;54(6):522–8.
17. Haissaguerre M, Derval N, Sacher F, et al. Sudden cardiac arrest associated with early repolarization. N Engl J Med 2008;358(19):2016–23.
18. Kataoka M, Takatsuki S, Tanimoto K, et al. A case of vagally mediated idiopathic ventricular fibrillation. Nat Clin Pract Cardiovasc Med 2008;5(2):111–5.
19. Kohsaka S, Razavi M, Massumi A. Idiopathic ventricular fibrillation successfully terminated by radiofrequency ablation of the distal Purkinje fibers. Pacing Clin Electrophysiol 2007;30(5):701–4.
20. Nogami A, Sugiyasu A, Kubota S, et al. Mapping and ablation of idiopathic ventricular fibrillation from the Purkinje system. Heart Rhythm 2005;2(6):646–9.
21. Saliba W, Abul Karim A, Tchou P, et al. Ventricular fibrillation: ablation of a trigger? J Cardiovasc Electrophysiol 2002;13(12):1296–9. Available at: http://onlinelibrary.wiley.com/doi/10.1046/j.1540-8167.2002.01296.x/abstract.
22. Takatsuki S, Mitamura H, Ogawa S. Catheter ablation of a monofocal premature ventricular complex triggering idiopathic ventricular fibrillation. Heart 2001;86(1):E3. Available at: http://www.ncbi.nlm.nih.gov/pmc/articles/PMC1729809/pdf/v086p000e3.pdf.
23. Yan GX, Antzelevitch C. Cellular basis for the Brugada syndrome and other mechanisms of

arrhythmogenesis associated with ST-segment elevation. Circulation 1999;100(15):1660–6. Available at: http://circ.ahajournals.org/content/100/15/1660.full.pdf.

24. Asano Y, Davidenko JM, Baxter WT, et al. Optical mapping of drug-induced polymorphic arrhythmias and torsade de pointes in the isolated rabbit heart. J Am Coll Cardiol 1997;29(4):831–42. Available at: http://ac.els-cdn.com/S0735109796005888/1-s2.0-S0735109796005888-main.pdf?_tid=a09cc1ec-9f5b-11e5-8bdf-00000aab0f6c&acdnat=1449765339_a80942bac5b519f93946e4587d19aaa8.

25. el-Sherif N, Caref EB, Yin H, et al. The electrophysiological mechanism of ventricular arrhythmias in the long QT syndrome. Tridimensional mapping of activation and recovery patterns. Circ Res 1996;79(3):474–92.

26. el-Sherif N, Zeiler RH, Craelius W, et al. QTU prolongation and polymorphic ventricular tachyarrhythmias due to bradycardia-dependent early afterdepolarizations. Afterdepolarizations and ventricular arrhythmias. Circ Res 1988;63(2):286–305. Available at: http://circres.ahajournals.org/content/63/2/286.full.pdf.

27. Haissaguerre M, Extramiana F, Hocini M, et al. Mapping and ablation of ventricular fibrillation associated with long-QT and Brugada syndromes. Circulation 2003;108(8):925–8.

28. Choi BR, Burton F, Salama G. Cytosolic Ca2+ triggers early afterdepolarizations and Torsade de Pointes in rabbit hearts with type 2 long QT syndrome. J Physiol 2002;543(Pt 2):615–31. Available at: http://www.ncbi.nlm.nih.gov/pmc/articles/PMC2290501/pdf/tjp0543-0615.pdf.

29. Tan VH, Yap J, Hsu LF, et al. Catheter ablation of ventricular fibrillation triggers and electrical storm. Europace 2012;14(12):1687–95.

30. Srivathsan K, Gami AS, Ackerman MJ, et al. Treatment of ventricular fibrillation in a patient with prior diagnosis of long QT syndrome: importance of precise electrophysiologic diagnosis to successfully ablate the trigger. Heart Rhythm 2007;4(8):1090–3.

31. Coronel R, Casini S, Koopmann TT, et al. Right ventricular fibrosis and conduction delay in a patient with clinical signs of Brugada syndrome: a combined electrophysiological, genetic, histopathologic,

and computational study. Circulation 2005;112(18):2769–77.

32. Darmon JP, Bettouche S, Deswardt P, et al. Radiofrequency ablation of ventricular fibrillation and multiple right and left atrial tachycardia in a patient with Brugada syndrome. J Interv Card Electrophysiol 2004;11(3):205–9.

33. Nakagawa E, Takagi M, Tatsumi H, et al. Successful radiofrequency catheter ablation for electrical storm of ventricular fibrillation in a patient with Brugada syndrome. Circ J 2008;72(6):1025–9. Available at: https://www.jstage.jst.go.jp/article/circj/72/6/72_6_1025/_pdf.

34. Nademanee K, Veerakul G, Chandanamattha P, et al. Prevention of ventricular fibrillation episodes in Brugada syndrome by catheter ablation over the anterior right ventricular outflow tract epicardium. Circulation 2011;123(12):1270–9.

35. Shah AJ, Hocini M, Lamaison D, et al. Regional substrate ablation abolishes Brugada syndrome. J Cardiovasc Electrophysiol 2011;22(11):1290–1.

36. Priori SG, Napolitano C, Tiso N, et al. Mutations in the cardiac ryanodine receptor gene (hRyR2) underlie catecholaminergic polymorphic ventricular tachycardia. Circulation 2001;103:196–200.

37. Leenhardt A, Lucet V, Denjoy I, et al. Catecholaminergic polymorphic ventricular tachycardia in children. A 7-year follow-up of 21 patients. Circulation 1995;91:1512–9.

38. Kaneshiro T, Naruse Y, Nogami A, et al. Successful catheter ablation of bidirectional ventricular premature contractions triggering ventricular fibrillation in catecholaminergic polymorphic ventricular tachycardia with RyR2 mutation. Circ Arrhythm Electrophysiol 2012;5(1):e14–7.

39. Giustetto C, Di Monte F, Wolpert C, et al. Short QT syndrome: clinical findings and diagnostic-therapeutic implications. Eur Heart J 2006;27(20):2440–7.

40. Yan GX, Antzelevitch C. Cellular basis for the electrocardiographic J wave. Circulation 1996;93(2):372–9.

41. Latcu DG, Bun SS, Zarqane N, et al. Ablation of left ventricular substrate in early repolarization syndrome. J Cardiovasc Electrophysiol 2016;27(4):490–1.

42. Umapathy K, Nair K, Masse S, et al. Phase mapping of cardiac fibrillation. Circ Arrhythm Electrophysiol 2010;3(1):105–14.

Exercise-induced Ventricular Tachycardia/ Ventricular Fibrillation in the Normal Heart

Risk Stratification and Management

Yoav Michowitz, MD, Sami Viskin, MD*, Raphael Rosso, MD

KEYWORDS

- Ventricular tachycardia • Ventricular fibrillation • Exercise
- Arrhythmogenic right ventricular cardiomyopathy • Mitral valve prolapse
- Catecholaminergic polymorphic ventricular tachycardia

KEY POINTS

- Ventricular tachycardia (VT) occurs only rarely in patients without organic heart disease, and most of these arrhythmic events are not related to exercise; consequently, the literature on exercise-induced VT/ventricular fibrillation in normal hearts is limited.
- The most common form of idiopathic monomorphic VT is the one originating from the outflow tract.
- The main point in risk stratification of exercise-induced monomorphic VT is distinguishing idiopathic monomorphic VT from VT related to subtle heart disease, particularly right ventricular dysplasia.
- Exercise-induced polymorphic VT is potentially lethal, particularly when caused by genetic disorders.

INTRODUCTION

Ventricular tachycardia (VT) and ventricular fibrillation (VF) occur only rarely in patients without organic heart disease, and most of these arrhythmic events are not related to exercise. Consequently, the literature on exercise-induced VT/VF in normal hearts is limited.[1–3] Idiopathic exercise-induced VT is rare even in the young population, in which organic heart disease is less common. For example, in a recent analysis of consecutive young (<18 years of age) patients treated for VT during a 25-year period, roughly half were free of organic heart disease and only half of these had exercise-induced VT.[4]

Furthermore, an arrhythmogenic genetic disorder was ultimately diagnosed in one-third of the patients with exercise-induced VT with apparently normal hearts.[4] Consequently, only 10 patients with exercise-induced idiopathic VT were identified during a 15-year period in a specialized referral center.[4] Analogously, among consecutive athletes undergoing evaluation for ventricular arrhythmias discovered during preparticipation screening, only 23% had persistence (9%) or worsening (14%) of arrhythmias during exercise; most had transient suppression of their ventricular arrhythmias during exercise, which reappeared during the recovery phase of the exercise test.[5] In addition, idiopathic VF is definitively rare and

Department of Cardiology, Tel Aviv Sourasky Medical Center, Sackler School of Medicine, Tel Aviv University, Weizman 6, Tel Aviv 64239, Israel
* Corresponding author.
E-mail address: samiviskin@gmail.com

Card Electrophysiol Clin 8 (2016) 593–600
http://dx.doi.org/10.1016/j.ccep.2016.04.008
1877-9182/16/$ – see front matter © 2016 Elsevier Inc. All rights reserved.

is not exercise related.[6,7] This article focuses on exercise-induced monomorphic (**Fig. 1**A) and polymorphic (**Fig. 1**B, C) VT in the absence of evident heart disease, with an emphasis on the differential diagnosis and its implications for risk stratification.

ARRHYTHMOGENIC EFFECTS OF EXERCISE

The mechanisms of ventricular arrhythmias in the normal heart are discussed (see Luebbert J, Auberson D, Marchlinski F: PVCs in Apparently Normal Hearts, in this issue). Exercise is arrhythmogenic, albeit causing mainly extrasystoles and nonsustained VT. The anticipation of dynamic exercise is associated with inhibition of vagal tone, increasing the sinus rate even before exercise begins.[8] Once exercise begins, the interplay between sympathetic activation and vagal withdrawal leads to increased heart rate and augmented ventricular contraction. In the postexercise phase, vagal reactivation decelerates the sinus rate, which may return to baseline within a few minutes while sympathetic tone is still increased. Sudden and unexpected exercise is associated with a different vagal withdrawn to sympathetic activation balance caused by earlier and more dramatic sympathetic activation.[8] Arrhythmogenic effects of exercise include shortening of the ventricular refractory periods, increased velocity of impulse conduction,

and enhanced amplitude of afterpotentials. All known mechanisms of cardiac arrhythmias (ie, reentry, triggered activity, and enhanced automaticity) play a role in the genesis of exercise-related arrhythmias.[8]

IDIOPATHIC MONOMORPHIC VENTRICULAR TACHYCARDIA

In its strictest form, the diagnosis of idiopathic VT should be reserved for patients with normal cardiac structure and function as assessed by noninvasive and invasive studies, including cardiac MRI, coronary angiography, ventriculography, and cardiac biopsy. However, in clinical practice, invasive evaluation is often voided when the clinical history and noninvasive studies suggest benign disease and the electrocardiogram (ECG) of the VT is consistent with well-described variants of idiopathic VT. Specific forms of VT often presenting in patients without apparent organic heart disease are presented in **Fig. 2**.[9] The most common form of idiopathic monomorphic VT (involving about 70% of idiopathic VT cases) originates from either the right ventricular outflow tract (RVOT) or the left ventricular outflow tract (LVOT). This form of VT is the ventricular arrhythmia most often encountered in otherwise healthy athletes.[10] The QRS morphology during VT is of left bundle branch block (LBBB) pattern with tall R waves in the

A

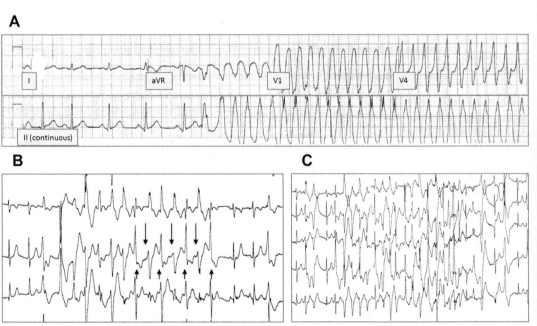

B

C

Fig. 1. Exercise-induced monomorphic and polymorphic VT. (*A*) A typical exercise-induced monomorphic VT. The arrhythmia is well tolerated despite its rapid rate. (*B*) The typical sequence of events recorded in patients with catecholamine-sensitive polymorphic VT. As the intensity of exercise increases, patients begin to develop more and more frequent ventricular ectopy and (if the exercise test continues) repetitive bursts of VT that may be bidirectional (*arrows in B*) and frankly polymorphic (*C*).

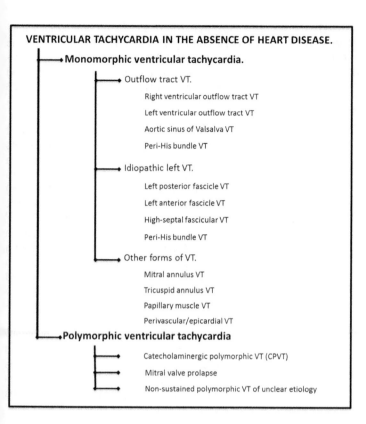

VENTRICULAR TACHYCARDIA IN THE ABSENCE OF HEART DISEASE.

→ Monomorphic ventricular tachycardia.

→ Outflow tract VT.

Right ventricular outflow tract VT

Left ventricular outflow tract VT

Aortic sinus of Valsalva VT

Peri-His bundle VT

→ Idiopathic left VT.

Left posterior fascicle VT

Left anterior fascicle VT

High-septal fascicular VT

Peri-His bundle VT

→ Other forms of VT.

Mitral annulus VT

Tricuspid annulus VT

Papillary muscle VT

Perivascular/epicardial VT

→ Polymorphic ventricular tachycardia

Catecholaminergic polymorphic VT (CPVT)

Mitral valve prolapse

Non-sustained polymorphic VT of unclear etiology

Fig. 2. Classification of ventricular tachycardia in the absence of heart disease based on morphology and site of origin. (*Adapted from* Prystowsky EN, Padanilam BJ, Joshi S, et al. Ventricular arrhythmias in the absence of structural heart disease. J Am Coll Cardiol 2012;59: 1733; with permission.)

inferior leads and normal or right axis.[11] Idiopathic outflow tract VT sometimes develops during exercise (usually in the form of salvos of repetitive exercise-induced VT)[12] but may also be suppressed by it, only to become sustained immediately after exercise (typically recorded during the recovery phase of an exercise test in susceptible patients).[13] It is generally considered a benign arrhythmia even when ventricular rates faster than 200 beats/min are recorded.

Idiopathic left ventricular (right bundle branch block pattern with mostly left-axis but rarely right-axis morphology) verapamil-responsive VT[14–16] is the second most common form of monomorphic idiopathic VT[7] and is rarely exercise induced.[17,18] Here too, the prognosis is good except for rare cases of tachycardia-induced cardiomyopathy.[7] Idiopathic VT originating from the papillary muscle is discussed (see Sung R, Scheinman M: Spectrum of Fascicular Arrhythmias, in this issue).

RISK STRATIFICATION AND MANAGEMENT

Idiopathic exercise-induced monomorphic VT is considered a benign arrhythmia. The authors[19]

and others[20] reported a malignant form of idiopathic RVOT-VT[21] leading to malignant syncope or cardiac arrest. However, this form of polymorphic VT is not exercise induced[19–21]; the malignant short-coupled variant of RVOT-VT is facilitated by vagal stimulation.[22] This form of idiopathic RVOT-VT is therefore not discussed here.

Cardiac arrest events have rarely been reported in cases with exercise-induced idiopathic monomorphic VT[7,23–25] but it is unclear whether these cases (reported years ago) involved truly idiopathic VT because cardiac MRI to exclude arrhythmogenic right ventricular cardiomyopathy (ARVC) was not always performed. Reported cases of apparently idiopathic RVOT-VT that resulted in fatalities ultimately had a diagnosis of ARVC confirmed only at autopsy.[26] Thus, a crucial step in the risk stratification process is deciding when a more aggressive evaluation is necessary for a case of apparently idiopathic VT to exclude the presence of unsuspected organic heart disease, which implicates higher risk of cardiac arrest. In particular, telling apart the rare cases of ARVC from the common cases of idiopathic RVOT-VT is both important and challenging.

MALIGNANT ARRHYTHMOGENIC RIGHT VENTRICULAR CARDIOMYOPATHY VERSUS BENIGN RIGHT VENTRICULAR OUTFLOW TRACT VENTRICULAR TACHYCARDIA

Distinguishing VT related to ARVC from the more common and benign RVOT-VT is critical because both forms present with ventricular arrhythmias with LBBB pattern.[27,28] This distinction is straightforward when ARVC is overt but may be challenging when not all the ECG features are present in patients with subtle forms of this inherited disorder.[27,28] For example, inverted T waves in V1 to V3 during sinus rhythm, one of the diagnostic criteria of ARVC, is present in only 32% of patients with ARVC and in 3% of healthy young individuals (and in a higher percentage of healthy children and adolescents).[29] Furthermore, the echocardiogram (normal by definition in idiopathic RVOT-VT), may miss as many as 50% of ARVC cases.[29]

In a study comparing ARVC-related VT with RVOT-VT,[28] the former showed wider QRS complexes in lead I during VT (150 ± 30 vs 123 ± 30 milliseconds; $P = .0006$) and more frequent QRS notching in at least 1 lead (65% vs 21%;

$P = .001$) than RVOT-VT.[28] Late precordial transition of R/S during VT (**Figs. 3** and **4**) was a specific characteristic of ARVC-related LBBB-VT (transition at V5 representing a 47% sensitivity and 90% specificity for ARVC-VT and transition at V6 representing an 18% sensitivity with 100% specificity).[28]

Important insights to the diagnosis of occult ARVC come from an important study of 30 patients with so-called silent ARVC, defined as carriers of a disease-causing ARVC mutation who were asymptomatic (at a mean age of 40 ± 19 years) and had normal ECG, normal echocardiogram, and normal or near-normal cardiac MRI.[30] Signal-averaged ECG detected late potentials in 36% of silent ARVC carriers. Furthermore, during exercise tests, new epsilon waves developed in 14% of ARVC carriers (but in none of the matched healthy controls; $P = .048$). In contrast, new T-wave inversion (observed only during or after exercise) had no diagnostic value.[30]

The documentation of fatal cases originally diagnosed as idiopathic RVOT-VT with eventual documentation of ARVC at autopsy raises the question of whether cardiac MRI should be performed in all patients with LBBB/inferior axis

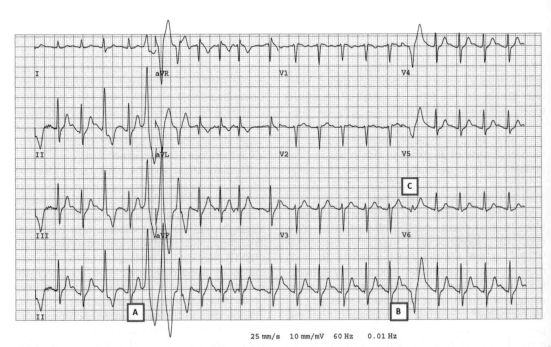

25 mm/s   10 mm/mV   60 Hz   0.01 Hz

Fig. 3. Exercise-induced ventricular arrhythmias in ARVC. Exercise-induced ventricular arrhythmias in a carrier of pathogenic ARVC mutation with no clinical manifestations of the disease who also had normal ECG, normal echocardiogram, and nondiagnostic cardiac MRI. Note that (1) the ventricular ectopy has more than 1 morphology (A vs B in continuous lead II), and (2) the ventricular ectopic beats with morphology have a late transition in the precordial leads (C). (*From* Perrin MJ, Angaran P, Laksman Z, et al. Exercise testing in asymptomatic gene carriers exposes a latent electrical substrate of arrhythmogenic right ventricular cardiomyopathy. J Am Coll Cardiol 2013;62:1772–9; with permission.)

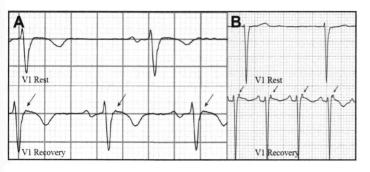

Fig. 4. Value of exercise test in ARVC in two different patients. Development of epsilon waves following exercise test in carriers of pathogenic ARVC mutation with no clinical manifestations of the disease who also had normal ECG, normal echocardiogram, and nondiagnostic cardiac MRI. Note that the epsilon waves are absent in the baseline ECG but are clearly seen in the recovery phase of an exercise test. (*From* Perrin MJ, Angaran P, Laksman Z, et al. Exercise testing in asymptomatic gene carriers exposes a latent electrical substrate of arrhythmogenic right ventricular cardiomyopathy. J Am Coll Cardiol 2013;62:1772–9; with permission.)

ectopy before the diagnosis of benign idiopathic RVOT-VT is accepted. In one series including 396 patients with greater than 1000 ventricular extrasystoles of apparent RVOT origin who had normal ECG and normal echocardiogram, almost one-third had abnormal cardiac MRI studies, including major and minor MRI abnormalities in 61 (15%) and 65 (16%) patients respectively.[31] Referral bias is one of the major concerns about this study because the high prevalence of these findings has not been confirmed by others. Although obtaining a cardiac MRI may not be necessary in every patient presenting with RVOT-VT and a normal echocardiogram, it should be considered in a high-risk subset, including patients with previous cardiac arrest, unexplained syncope, and rapid or polymorphic VT. VT (as opposed to only frequent extrasystoles) was more likely to be recorded among patients with abnormal MRI.[31] Moreover, the risk of serious arrhythmic events (sudden death, cardiac arrest of implantable cardioverter-defibrillator [ICD] shock) was significantly higher (hazard ratio of 27, 95% confidence interval 3–244) for patients older than 20 years who had cardiac MRI abnormalities.[31] The mode of VT induction during electrophysiologic studies (programmed ventricular extrastimulation vs burst pacing or isoproterenol infusion) also helps in distinguishing ARVC from idiopathic VT cases because VT is caused by reentry in ARVC but by enhanced automaticity in idiopathic RVOT-VT.[32]

EXERCISE-INDUCED VENTRICULAR TACHYCARDIA AND BRUGADA SYNDROME

Worsening of the electrocardiographic manifestations of Brugada syndrome (ie, augmentation of the ST segment elevation) may occur during[33] or immediately after[34] exercise. The latter finding is associated with higher arrhythmic risk during long-term follow-up,[34] but not with exercise-induced arrhythmias. The authors have encountered only 1 patient with Brugada syndrome who had exercise-induced sustained monomorphic VT.[35] This sustained monomorphic VT was detected during an exercise test evaluation after cardiac arrest.[36] Here too, the only clinical arrhythmias detected by the patient's implanted defibrillator, over years of follow-up, were polymorphic VT spontaneously occurring during sleep.[36]

The fact that fever is a well-recognized trigger of arrhythmias in Brugada syndrome[37,38] has raised concerns that some cases of exercise-induced heat stroke presenting with unheralded cardiac arrest[39] could be caused by heat-induced arrhythmias from Brugada syndrome. Also, monomorphic VT is a rare manifestation of Brugada syndrome (seen mainly in children)[40] and is almost never provoked by exercise. Consequently, avoidance of exercise is not listed among the recommended lifestyle modifications for patients with Brugada syndrome according to present guidelines.[41] However, because enhanced vagal tone is proarrhythmic in Brugada syndrome[36] the authors recommend that patients with Brugada syndrome avoid sudden termination of strenuous exercise that could trigger a vagal response.

EXERCISE-INDUCED POLYMORPHIC VENTRICULAR TACHYCARDIA

Catecholamine-sensitive polymorphic VT (CPVT) is a genetic disorder caused by mutations in the following genes: RyR2, CASQ2, and rarely KCNJ2, Ank2, TRDN, and CALM1.[41] It manifests clinically as arrhythmic syncope or cardiac arrest, characteristically occurring during physical or emotional stress. Patients with CPVT generally show atrial and ventricular arrhythmias during exercise, including atrial fibrillation. As the level of exercise increases, frequent ventricular ectopy (often resembling RVO-VT ectopy)[42] is succeeded by repetitive nonsustained VT that is either bidirectional or frankly polymorphic (see **Fig. 1**B, C).[7] CPVT is a highly malignant disease: roughly 60% of patients develop malignant syncope or cardiac arrest within a decade of diagnosis if left untreated.[43] β-Blocker therapy is mandatory even for silent carriers (patients with identified mutations but negative exercise test) because cardiac arrest may be the presenting symptom in such patients.[44] Also, β-blocker therapy reduces by half the long-term risk of recurrent exercise-induced arrhythmias. However, even this 30% residual risk of serious arrhythmic events (on β-blocker therapy)[44] is unacceptably high. Therefore, additional therapy with flecainide[45] and left cardiac sympathetic denervation[46] are strongly recommended for patients who have recurrence of symptoms or evidence of exercise-induced ventricular ectopy on β-blocker therapy during repeated exercise tests. ICD implantation is not recommended as stand-alone therapy because ICD shocks can trigger arrhythmic storms that can be lethal.[41] The ICD is recommended for patients who experience symptoms despite optimal therapy (β-blockers, flecainide, and left cardiac sympathetic denervation).[41]

Arrhythmias similar to those recorded in CPVT (including bidirectional and polymorphic VT) may be recorded in the Andersen-Tawil syndrome caused by KCNJ2 mutations.[47] As opposed to patients with CPVT, patients with Andersen-Tawil have frequent arrhythmias at rest and generally (but not invariably)[48,49] have a better prognosis.

Exercise-induced polymorphic VT (usually repetitive short bursts) is recorded in a minority of patients with mitral valve prolapse (MVP). MVP accounts for 7% of sudden death cases in the young population (13% of sudden death cases among young female patients).[50] Clinical and ECG characteristics associated with increased risk for sudden death in MVP include (1) female gender, (2) biphasic or inverted T waves in the inferolateral leads, (3) high burden of ventricular ectopy (usually multifocal or alternating [papillary muscle–LVOT origin] and nonsustained VT).[50,51]

Exercise-induced nonsustained polymorphic VT has been associated with digitalis toxicity and with myocarditis.[52] Exercise-induced polymorphic VT deteriorating to VF may occur during exercise-induced acute myocardial infarction. In addition, short bursts of exercise-induced polymorphic VT may be recorded in patients with stable coronary disease and also in healthy athletes. In such cases, the arrhythmia is usually not reproducible during repeated exercise tests. In such cases, the authors empirically recommend β-blocker therapy. If coronary artery disease is suspected, a coronary angiogram should be performed, especially in the presence of ischemia documented by imaging or electrocardiography.

SUMMARY/DISCUSSION

Exercise-induced VT only rarely occurs in the absence of organic heart disease. Idiopathic monomorphic VT has an excellent prognosis even if the VT rate is fast. The main aspect of the risk stratification process is recognizing the presence of subtle forms of organic heart disease, particularly ARVC. Characteristics that favor ARVC more than idiopathic VT of LBBB pattern include wider or notched QRS complexes, with a late R/S transition in the precordial leads during VT. Exercise-induced polymorphic VT is potentially malignant. In CPVT, provocation of bidirectional and polymorphic VT reproducibly occurs during increasing levels of exercise. Exercise-induced polymorphic VT has also been seen in MVP. Some patients with stable coronary disease, and even healthy athletes, sometimes have short bursts of polymorphic VT during exercise test but these arrhythmias are usually not reproducible during repeated testing and have unknown long-term clinical significance.

REFERENCES

1. Mont L, Seixas T, Brugada P, et al. The electrocardiographic, clinical, and electrophysiologic spectrum of idiopathic monomorphic ventricular tachycardia. Am Heart J 1992;124:746–53.
2. Mont L, Seixas T, Brugada P, et al. Clinical and electrophysiologic characteristics of exercise-related idiopathic ventricular tachycardia. Am J Cardiol 1991;68:897–900.
3. Palileo EV, Ashley WW, Swiryn S, et al. Exercise provocable right ventricular outflow tract tachycardia. Am Heart J 1982;104:185–93.
4. Wang S, Zhu W, Hamilton RM, et al. Diagnosis-specific characteristics of ventricular tachycardia in children with structurally normal hearts. Heart Rhythm 2010;7:1725–31.
5. Steriotis AK, Nava A, Rigato I, et al. Noninvasive cardiac screening in young athletes with ventricular arrhythmias. Am J Cardiol 2013;111:557–62.
6. Viskin S, Belhassen B. Idiopathic ventricular fibrillation. Am Heart J 1990;120:661–71.
7. Belhassen B, Viskin S. Idiopathic ventricular tachycardia and fibrillation. J Cardiovasc Electrophysiol 1993;4:356–68.

8. Balady G, Morise AP. Exercise testing. In: Mann DL, Zipes DP, Libby P, et al, editors. Braunwald's heart disease: a textbook of cardiovascular medicine. 10th edition. Philadelphia: Elsevier/Saunders; 2015.

9. Prystowsky EN, Padanilam BJ, Joshi S, et al. Ventricular arrhythmias in the absence of structural heart disease. J Am Coll Cardiol 2012;59:1733–44.

10. Biffi A, Pelliccia A, Verdile L, et al. Long-term clinical significance of frequent and complex ventricular tachyarrhythmias in trained athletes. J Am Coll Cardiol 2002;40:446–52.

11. Buxton AE, Waxman HL, Marchlinski FE, et al. Right ventricular tachycardia: clinical and electrophysiologic characteristics. Circulation 1983;68:917–27.

12. Wu D, Kou HC, Hung JS. Exercise-triggered paroxysmal ventricular tachycardia. A repetitive rhythmic activity possibly related to afterdepolarization. Ann Intern Med 1981;95:410–4.

13. Kienzle MG, Martins JB, Constantin L, et al. Effect of direct, reflex and exercise-provoked increases in sympathetic tone on idiopathic ventricular tachycardia. Am J Cardiol 1992;69:1433–8.

14. Belhassen B, Rotmensch HH, Laniado S. Response of recurrent sustained ventricular tachycardia to verapamil. Br Heart J 1981;46:679–82.

15. Belhassen B, Shapira I, Pelleg A, et al. Idiopathic recurrent sustained ventricular tachycardia responsive to verapamil: an ECG-electrophysiologic entity. Am Heart J 1984;108:1034–7.

16. Zipes DP, Foster PR, Troup PJ, et al. Atrial induction of ventricular tachycardia: reentry versus triggered automaticity. Am J Cardiol 1979;44:1–8.

17. Klein GJ, Millman PJ, Yee R. Recurrent ventricular tachycardia responsive to verapamil. Pacing Clin Electrophysiol 1984;7:938–48.

18. Sung RJ, Shapiro WA, Shen EN, et al. Effects of verapamil on ventricular tachycardias possibly caused by reentry, automaticity, and triggered activity. J Clin Invest 1983;72:350–60.

19. Viskin S, Rosso R, Rogowski O, et al. The "short-coupled" variant of right ventricular outflow ventricular tachycardia: a not-so-benign form of benign ventricular tachycardia? J Cardiovasc Electrophysiol 2005;16:912–6.

20. Noda T, Shimizu W, Taguchi A, et al. Malignant entity of idiopathic ventricular fibrillation and polymorphic ventricular tachycardia initiated by premature extrasystoles originating from the right ventricular outflow tract. J Am Coll Cardiol 2005;46:1288–94.

21. Shimizu W. Arrhythmias originating from the right ventricular outflow tract: how to distinguish "malignant" from "benign"? Heart Rhythm 2009;6: 1507–11.

22. Kataoka M, Takatsuki S, Tanimoto K, et al. A case of vagally mediated idiopathic ventricular fibrillation. Nat Clin Pract Cardiovasc Med 2008;5:111–5.

23. James TN, MacLean WA. Paroxysmal ventricular arrhythmias and familial sudden death associated with neural lesions in the heart. Chest 1980;78: 24–30.

24. Miller SM, Martinez JJ, Deal BJ, et al. Electrophysiologic testing of tocainide and mexiletine for ventricular tachycardia: assessment of the need to test both drugs. Am Heart J 1986;112:1114–6.

25. Rowland TW, Schweiger MJ. Repetitive paroxysmal ventricular tachycardia and sudden death in a child. Am J Cardiol 1984;53:1729.

26. Tada H, Ohe T, Yutani C, et al. Sudden death in a patient with apparent idiopathic ventricular tachycardia. Jpn Circ J 1996;60:133–6.

27. Hoffmayer KS, Bhave PD, Marcus GM, et al. An electrocardiographic scoring system for distinguishing right ventricular outflow tract arrhythmias in patients with arrhythmogenic right ventricular cardiomyopathy from idiopathic ventricular tachycardia. Heart Rhythm 2013;10:477–82.

28. Hoffmayer KS, Machado ON, Marcus GM, et al. Electrocardiographic comparison of ventricular arrhythmias in patients with arrhythmogenic right ventricular cardiomyopathy and right ventricular outflow tract tachycardia. J Am Coll Cardiol 2011; 58:831–8.

29. Marcus FI, Zareba W, Calkins H, et al. Arrhythmogenic right ventricular cardiomyopathy/dysplasia clinical presentation and diagnostic evaluation: results from the North American Multidisciplinary Study. Heart Rhythm 2009;6:984–92.

30. Perrin MJ, Angaran P, Laksman Z, et al. Exercise testing in asymptomatic gene carriers exposes a latent electrical substrate of arrhythmogenic right ventricular cardiomyopathy. J Am Coll Cardiol 2013;62:1772–9.

31. Aquaro GD, Pingitore A, Strata E, et al. Cardiac magnetic resonance predicts outcome in patients with premature ventricular complexes of left bundle branch block morphology. J Am Coll Cardiol 2010; 56:1235–43.

32. O'Donnell D, Cox D, Bourke J, et al. Clinical and electrophysiological differences between patients with arrhythmogenic right ventricular dysplasia and right ventricular outflow tract tachycardia. Eur Heart J 2003;24:801–10.

33. Amin AS, de Groot EA, Ruijter JM, et al. Exercise-induced ECG changes in Brugada syndrome. Circ Arrhythm Electrophysiol 2009;2:531–9.

34. Makimoto H, Nakagawa E, Takaki H, et al. Augmented ST-segment elevation during recovery from exercise predicts cardiac events in patients with Brugada syndrome. J Am Coll Cardiol 2010; 56:1576–84.

35. Viskin S, Belhassen B. Clinical problem solving: when you only live twice. N Engl J Med 1995;332: 1221–5.

36. Adler A, Rosso R, Chorin E, et al. Risk stratification in Brugada syndrome: clinical characteristics, electrocardiographic parameters, and auxiliary testing. Heart Rhythm 2016;13(1):299–310.

37. Adler A, Topaz G, Heller K, et al. Fever induced type I Brugada pattern: how common is it and what does this mean? Heart Rhythm 2013;10(9):1375–82.

38. Keller DI, Rougier JS, Kucera JP, et al. Brugada syndrome and fever: genetic and molecular characterization of patients carrying SCN5A mutations. Cardiovasc Res 2005;67:510–9.

39. Yankelson L, Sadeh B, Gershovitz L, et al. Life-threatening events during endurance sports: is heat stroke more prevalent than arrhythmic death? J Am Coll Cardiol 2014;64:463–9.

40. Probst V, Denjoy I, Meregalli PG, et al. Clinical aspects and prognosis of Brugada syndrome in children. Circulation 2007;115:2042–8.

41. Priori SG, Wilde AA, Horie M, et al. HRS/EHRA/APHRS expert consensus statement on the diagnosis and management of patients with inherited primary arrhythmia syndromes. Heart Rhythm 2013;10:1932–63.

42. Sumitomo N, Harada K, Nagashima M, et al. Catecholaminergic polymorphic ventricular tachycardia: electrocardiographic characteristics and optimal therapeutic strategies to prevent sudden death. Heart 2003;89:66–70.

43. Leenhardt A, Denjoy I, Guicheney P. Catecholaminergic polymorphic ventricular tachycardia. Circ Arrhythm Electrophysiol 2012;5:1044–52.

44. Hayashi M, Denjoy I, Extramiana F, et al. Incidence and risk factors of arrhythmic events in catecholaminergic polymorphic ventricular tachycardia. Circulation 2009;119:2426–34.

45. van der Werf C, Kannankeril PJ, Sacher F, et al. Flecainide therapy reduces exercise-induced ventricular arrhythmias in patients with catecholaminergic polymorphic ventricular tachycardia. J Am Coll Cardiol 2011;57:2244–54.

46. Collura CA, Johnson JN, Moir C, et al. Left cardiac sympathetic denervation for the treatment of long QT syndrome and catecholaminergic polymorphic ventricular tachycardia using video-assisted thoracic surgery. Heart Rhythm 2009;6:752–9.

47. Miyamoto K, Aiba T, Kimura H, et al. Efficacy and safety of flecainide for ventricular arrhythmias in patients with Andersen-Tawil syndrome with KCNJ2 mutations. Heart Rhythm 2015;12:596–603.

48. Efremidis M, Pappas LK, Sideris A, et al. Swimming-triggered aborted sudden cardiac death in a patient with Andersen-Tawil syndrome. Int J Cardiol 2006; 112:e45–47.

49. Fernlund E, Lundin C, Hertervig E, et al. Novel mutation in the KCNJ2 gene is associated with a malignant arrhythmic phenotype of Andersen-Tawil syndrome. Ann Noninvasive Electrocardiol 2013; 18:471–8.

50. Basso C, Perazzolo Marra M, Rizzo S, et al. Arrhythmic mitral valve prolapse and sudden cardiac death. Circulation 2015;132:556–66.

51. Sriram CS, Syed FF, Ferguson ME, et al. Malignant bileaflet mitral valve prolapse syndrome in patients with otherwise idiopathic out-of-hospital cardiac arrest. J Am Coll Cardiol 2013;62:222–30.

52. van der Werf C, Wilde AA. Catecholaminergic polymorphic ventricular tachycardia: from bench to bedside. Heart 2013;99:497–504.

Dynamics and Molecular Mechanisms of Ventricular Fibrillation in Structurally Normal Hearts

José Jalife, MD

KEYWORDS

- Rotors • Dominant frequency • Fibrillatory conduction ionic mechanisms
- Na$_V$1.5-Kir2.1 interactions

KEY POINTS

- Ventricular fibrillation (VF) is an important immediate cause of sudden cardiac death.
- VF is driven by a small number (1 or 2) of high-frequency rotors that generate spiral waves whose fragmentation in the periphery of the rotor give rise to the complex patterns of activation that are known as fibrillatory conduction.
- The interbeat interval of VF scales as body mass$^{1/4}$ indicating that there is a strong similarity in the underlying mechanisms of VF in all mammalian species, including humans.
- At the molecular level, the frequency and complexity of the rotors that maintain VF depend on the expression, spatial distribution, and intermolecular interactions of the inward rectifier potassium channel, Kir2.1, and the alpha subunit of the main cardiac sodium channel, Na$_V$1.5.

INTRODUCTION

Ventricular fibrillation (VF) is an important immediate cause of sudden cardiac death, which is a major global public health problem accounting for an estimated 15% to 20% of all deaths.[1] Epidemiologic studies from the 1970s through the 1990s suggested that 88% to 91% of deaths that occur within 1 hour of symptom onset were arrhythmic in nature, presumably VF.[2] During VF, the sequence of ventricular activation is extremely abnormal and electrical impulses do not follow the usual paths.[3] The heart rate accelerates to the extreme, and the electrical waves assume a complex vortexlike behavior that brings to mind eddy formation and turbulence in water.[4] Turbulent excitation produces uncoordinated contraction, which renders the heart unable to pump blood. Thus, the blood pressure decreases, immediate loss of consciousness follows, and death is near unless a defibrillating shock is applied. This article reviews the current understanding of the dynamics of wave propagation and the molecular mechanisms underlying VF in the structurally normal mammalian heart. Particular attention is given to the dynamics of self-organization of cardiac electrical waves into the high-frequency rotors that result in fibrillatory conduction and the role of 2 major cardiac ion channels responsible for cardiac excitability in the underlying mechanism of rotor formation and VF maintenance.

Disclosure: The author has nothing to disclose.
This work was supported in part by the National Heart, Lung, and Blood Institute R01 (HL122352) NIH/NHLBI, and the Leducq Foundation: Transatlantic Network of Excellence Program on Structural Alterations in the Myocardium and the Substrate for Cardiac Fibrillation.
Center for Arrhythmia Research, North Campus Research Complex, University of Michigan, 2800 Plymouth Road, Ann Arbor, MI 48109, USA
E-mail address: jjalife@umich.edu

MODERN CONCEPTS ON VENTRICULAR FIBRILLATION MECHANISMS

On electrocardiogram (ECG), VF is characterized by the presence of highly irregular QRS complexes of varying morphology, amplitude, and frequency. Traditionally, such an apparently aperiodic and irregular activation of the ventricles was interpreted as being totally disorganized,[5,6] which led to the idea that VF was the result of a continuous self-sustaining activation by multiple wavelets that propagated randomly throughout the ventricles.[6] In the 1970s and 1980s, a new idea began to emerge based on theoretic[7,8] and experimental[9] findings, which showed that the heart could sustain electrical activity that rotated about a functional obstacle. Such "rotors" were thought to be the major organizing centers of fibrillation. Since then, several studies have focused on rotors as the underlying mechanism for ventricular tachycardia (VT) and VF in the heart. However, 2 schools of thought emerged. Many of the proposed mechanisms for fibrillation focused on fleetingness and instability of rotors,[10,11] and for some time substantial experimental[12–14] and theoretic work[15] accumulated suggesting that turbulence in VF is associated with breakup of a single spiral wave or a pair of counter-rotating spiral waves into a multispiral disordered state.[11]

However, alternative explanations for the breakup of the rotor in the three-dimensional myocardium have been proposed. One such mechanism, referred to as the restitution hypothesis, suggests that the breakup of the rotor into a multispiral state ensues when the oscillations of the action potential duration (APD) are of sufficiently large amplitude to cause block of conduction along the wave front.[16] The idea built on previous work showing that the slope of the electrical restitution relation determines certain dynamical behavior that may be conducive to the development of VF.[17] In particular, if the slope of the action potential restitution curve, in which duration of the action potential is plotted against the preceding diastolic interval, is greater than 1, then APD alternans is possible.[17] The initiation of APD alternans was proposed to be the first step in period-doubling sequences that culminate in complex behavior.[18–20] Subsequently, this process resulted in the destabilization of the wave fronts and the formation of a multispiral state.[12] Another mechanism for breakup focused on the highly anisotropic, rotational, and layered nature of the fibers of the three-dimensional ventricular myocardium, which produces twisting and instability of the organizing center (filament), and results in its multiplication following repeated collisions with boundaries in the heart.[21]

Over the past 25 years, work from my laboratory has focused on rotors as the primary engines of fibrillation.[22–25] However, in contrast with the breakup mechanism of VF, we proposed that VF was a problem of self-organization of nonlinear electrical waves with both deterministic and stochastic components.[4,24] Our studies strongly supported and continue to support the hypothesis that, in the structurally normal heart, there is both spatial and temporal organization during VF, although there is a wide spectrum of behavior.[26] On one end, we showed that a single drifting rotor could give rise to a complex pattern of excitation that was reminiscent of VF.[24] On the other end, we showed that VF could also be driven by a highly stable high-frequency source and that the complex patterns of activation were the result of the fragmentation of spiral electrical waves emanating from that source (ie, fibrillatory conduction).[27,28]

FIBRILLATORY CONDUCTION

Gray and colleagues[24] showed unequivocally that, in the rabbit heart, even a single drifting rotor can produce an ECG that is indistinguishable from VF. However, it has also been shown that in other mammalian hearts a more complex spatiotemporal organization may prevail. This finding led us to suggest that some forms of fibrillation depend on the uninterrupted periodic activity of discrete reentrant circuits.[27,29] As shown in the computer simulation of VF presented in **Fig. 1**, the faster rotors act as the dominant frequency (DF) sources, which maintain the overall activity. The rapidly succeeding wave fronts emanating from such sources propagate throughout the ventricles and interact with tissue heterogeneities, functional and anatomic, leading to fragmentation and wavelet formation.[3,23] The newly formed wavelets may undergo decremental conduction or they may be annihilated by collision with another wavelet or a boundary, and still others may form new sustained rotors. Thus, the result would be fibrillatory conduction or the frequency-dependent fragmentation of wave fronts, emanating from high-frequency reentrant circuits, into multiple independent wavelets.[27,30]

Using spectral analysis of optical epicardial and endocardial signals for sheep ventricular slabs, Zaitsev and colleagues[31] provided additional evidence suggesting that rotors and fibrillatory conduction may be the underlying mechanism of VF. The data showed that the DFs of excitation (ie, peak with maximal power) do not change continuously on the ventricular surfaces of slabs[31]; the frequencies are constant over regions termed domains. Moreover, there

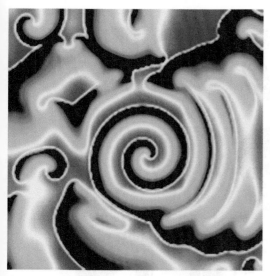

Fig. 1. Rotor and fibrillatory conduction in a computer simulation. The rotor is the driver of reentry that lies at the center of a spiral wave; its spinning rate determines the degree of turbulence (fractionation) around it: The higher the spinning rate, the greater the amount of fractionation. Rotors as drivers are not easy to find: in this computer simulation the so-called mother rotor occupies less than 0.1 of the medium. The rest is fibrillatory conduction.

are only a small number of discrete domains found on the ventricular surfaces. They also showed that the DFs of excitation in the adjacent domains were often 1:2, 3:4, or 4:5 ratios of the fastest DF domain and this was suggested to be the result of intermittent Wenckebach-like conduction blocks at the boundaries between domains.[31] Thus, they concluded that VF may be the result of a sustained high-frequency three-dimensional intramural scroll wave, which creates a highly complex pattern of activation when wave fronts emanating from it fragment as the result of interaction with the heterogeneities present in the cardiac tissue.[31]

SCALING LAW OF VENTRICULAR FIBRILLATION FREQUENCY

Based on normal electrophysiology and anatomy, Schmidt-Nielsen[32] suggested that all mammalian hearts are built on the same template, and fibrillation has been shown to occur in the hearts of all mammalian species studied to date, from the mouse to the horse.[33] The question therefore arises as to whether the spatiotemporal properties of VF scale with body mass (BM). More specifically, are rotors spinning at high frequency the universal mechanism of sudden death caused by

VF. Several years ago my laboratory investigated whether the temporal properties of VF, the major cause of sudden and unexpected cardiac death, scale with BM.[33] By using high-resolution optical mapping, numerical simulations, and meta-analysis of VF data in 11 mammalian species, we showed that the interbeat interval of VF scales as VF cycle length = $53 \times BM^{1/4}$, spanning more than 4 orders of magnitude in BM from mouse to horse.[33] Fibrillatory behavior is shown by the data in **Fig. 2**, which were obtained by high-resolution optical mapping of Langendorff-perfused hearts from 4 different mammals (mouse, guinea pig, sheep, and human). We used a fluorescent voltage-sensitive dye and a charge-coupled device (CCD) camera that was focused on the anterior ventricular surface. Snapshots taken from phase movies of wave-propagation dynamics during stable VF revealed sustained rotors whose rotation frequency depended on the species (mouse, 38 Hz; guinea pig, 26 Hz; sheep, 12 Hz; human, 6.8 Hz). Therefore, although the understanding of the molecular mechanisms of fatal arrhythmias such as VF from small mammals to humans is still incomplete, our demonstration that the interbeat interval of VF scales as $BM^{1/4}$ suggests that there might be a strong similarity in the underlying mechanisms of VF in most, if not all, mammalian species, including humans, which may be of considerable fundamental and clinical significance.[33]

THE GUINEA PIG HEART MODEL OF VENTRICULAR FIBRILLATION

In 2001, we presented evidence in the isolated guinea pig heart that strongly supported the hypothesis that fibrillatory conduction from a stable high-frequency rotor is the underlying mechanism of VF in this species.[34] Using a high-resolution CCD video camera, optical recordings of potentiometric dye fluorescence from the epicardial ventricular surface were obtained along with a volume-conducted global ECG. Transmembrane signals at each pixel location showed a strong periodic component centered near 12 Hz on the anterior surface of the left ventricle (LV) with turbulent activity (fibrillatory conduction) toward the rest of the anterior and posterior surfaces of the LV and the right ventricle (RV; **Fig. 3**). This periodicity was seen as an attractor in two-dimensional-phase space and each site could be represented by its phase around the attractor.[25] As shown in **Fig. 3A**, spatial phase maps of the anterior and posterior ventricular surfaces at each instant revealed the source of fibrillation in the form of a phase singularity (a rotor) on the anterior surface of the LV. In **Fig. 3B**, spectral analysis of

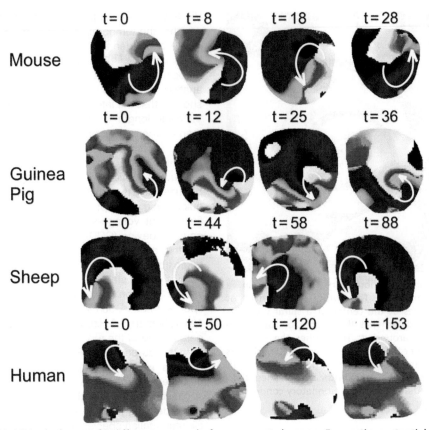

Fig. 2. Stable VF in the hearts of 4 different mammals, from mouse to humans. Four action-potential-phase snap-shots depict a rotation of spirals in mouse, guinea pig, sheep, and human hearts. Vortexlike reentry is apparent in all hearts. The white curved arrows mark the location of the center and the direction of rotation. Numbers above each map represent time in milliseconds after an arbitrary zero. (*Adapted from* Noujaim SF, Berenfeld O, Kalifa J, et al. Universal scaling law of electrical turbulence in the mammalian heart. Proc Natl Acad Sci U S A 2007;104:20985–9; with permission.)

optical signals (pixel by pixel) revealed that DFs were distributed throughout the ventricles in clearly demarcated domains.[27] The highest frequency domains were always found on the anterior wall of the LV. Moreover, optical data showed wave breaks and conduction blocks in the periphery of the high-frequency domains. Thus, the results showed that, in the isolated guinea pig heart, a high-frequency reentrant source that remained stationary in the LV was the mechanism that sustained VF.[27]

ACTION POTENTIAL DURATION ABBREVIATION AND RAPID ROTATION FREQUENCY

During VF the activation rate is significantly faster than that achievable by either pacemaker activity or rapid pacing.[35,36] Similarly, in our experiments rotors achieved cycle lengths (CLs; ~30–40 milliseconds) that were significantly briefer than expected from the guinea pig heart, in which APD is typically ~200 milliseconds at

1 Hz.[37] Computer simulations suggested that the activation at extremely fast rates by rotors is the result of the strong repolarizing influence exerted by their core, which abbreviates the APD in its proximity. However, with increasing distance from the core, this influence weakens and the APD progressively increases.[38] Consequently, the tissue close to the core achieves very fast CLs, whereas, far from the core, the myocardium could not be excited at the rate of the rotor and nonuniform (ie, other than 1:1) conduction developed.[39] In theory, this effect may provide a basis for the gradient in DFs observed in the guinea pig ventricles during VF (see **Fig. 3**B). Propagation near the rotor is usually 1:1; however, at a certain distance from the rotor, conduction blocks and wave breaks develop and slower DF domains are formed.[27,34] Nevertheless, although this mechanism may account for the shortening of the APD and the formation of DF domains, it does not explain the consistent localization of the fastest DF domain to the anterior free wall of the LV.

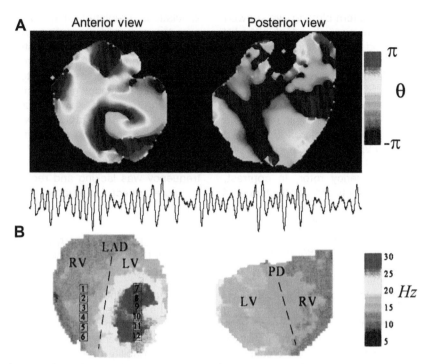

Fig. 3. (*A, top*) A snapshot of a spatial color phase map of the anterior and posterior ventricular surfaces at each instant during ventricular fibrillation reveals a rotor on the anterior surface of the LV, with fibrillatory conduction to the rest of the ventricles. (*Bottom*) ECG during VF. (*B*) Quantification of DF maps. (*A*) Mean DF maps constructed from 9 experiments. Left, anterior view; right, posterior view. (*B*) Maps of the standard devition of the DFs. Left, anterior view; right, posterior view. See text for further details. LAD, left anterior descending artery; PD, posterior descending artery. (*Adapted from* Samie FH, Mandapati R, Gray RA, et al. A mechanism of transition from ventricular fibrillation to tachycardia: effect of calcium channel blockade on the dynamics of rotating waves. Circ Res 2000;86:684–91; with permission.)

Answering that question required the use of the whole-cell patch-clamp technique and computer simulations, which showed that regional differences in the distribution of an inward rectifier potassium channel provided an ionic mechanism for the localization of the source in the LV and the establishment of a consistent gradient of excitation frequency between the LV and the RV during VF.[34]

AN IONIC MECHANISM FOR STABLE ROTORS AND VENTRICULAR FIBRILLATION

The fact that the driving rotor was confined to a small area of the LV of the fibrillating guinea pig heart[34] strongly supported the so-called mother rotor hypothesis.[28,30] The finding was nevertheless surprising at the time and required a detailed mechanistic explanation because everyone in this field knew that the anatomic structure of the ventricles was highly heterogeneous, and was intuitively more likely to contribute to breakup rather than stability. However, what if the specific structural heterogeneity of the

ventricles contributes to rotor confinement? One form of heterogeneity that had not been discovered was that the background potassium current of the cells in the RV was different from that in the LV. The dominant component of such a current in ventricular myocytes is the inward rectifier potassium current (I_{K1}) carried primarily by Kir2.1 channels. I_{K1} contributes a large inward conductance at membrane potentials less than the potassium equilibrium potential (E_K), which together with the large outward conductance at potentials slightly greater than E_K helps maintain the ventricular resting membrane potential at approximately −85 mV.[40] In addition, I_{K1} is an important determinant of cardiac excitability and helps control the APD by contributing outward current during the final phase of repolarization.[41,42]

Computer simulations suggested that rotor stability in the LV resulted from a large repolarizing outward current that hastened repolarization and shortened APD, whereas instability, termination, and wave breaks in the RV were a consequence of strong rectification and longer APD.[34] Using reverse transcription polymerase chain reaction and Western blotting, we showed that Kir2.1 proteins are more abundant in the LV than in the RV,[43] and patch-clamp experiments confirmed that the outward component in the current-voltage relation of I_{K1} was larger in the LV than in the RV.[34,43] As shown in **Fig. 4**A, B, on incorporating the ionic current values derived from experimental data into our ionic model, we observed that the large outward conductance of I_{K1}, simulating the LV, produced the necessary abbreviation of the APD for the establishment of a stable high-frequency rotor. In contrast, the model with small outward conductance of I_{K1}, simulating the RV, was unable to sustain a rotor because the wave front and wave tail collided, trapped the tip of the rotor, and thus terminated the activity. Moreover, when LV and RV models were coupled in a two-dimensional sheet, the numerical results accurately reproduced the experimental VF data (**Fig. 4**C, D). Under these conditions, the high-frequency rotor in the LV became the engine that maintained the overall activity in both ventricles, with the RV producing multiple short-lived wave breaks and nonsustained reentry whose intrinsic frequency was much slower than in the LV.[34] Thus, our

simulations predicted that, by reducing APD near the core and preventing wave front–wave tail interactions, the larger amplitude of the outward component of I_{K1} in LV myocytes should stabilize the high-frequency rotor in the LV.[34] Moreover, pharmacologic reduction of I_{K1} density using $BaCl_2$ at low concentrations was shown to terminate stable VF, which supported a role of this current in rotor dynamics.[43] However, direct proof for the role of inward rectifier channels in the control of rotor stability and frequency was lacking and required the use of a more direct approach involving mouse genetics.

MOUSE GENETICS, INWARD RECTIFIER POTASSIUM CURRENT AND VENTRICULAR FIBRILLATION

Genetically engineered mice are valuable tools in which the electrophysiologic consequences of genetic manipulation of ion channels can be directly determined. Several years ago we took advantage of the availability of a transgenic (TG) mouse in which I_{K1} was upregulated by overexpressing the Kir2.1 protein in the heart under control of the

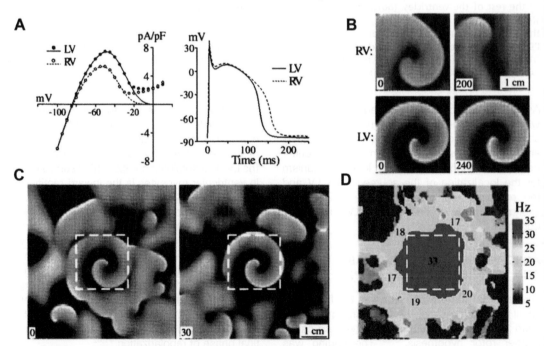

Fig. 4. Computer simulations. (*A*) Formulation of I_{K1} used in the model (*solid and broken lines*) with corresponding action potentials. Mean experimental data from **Fig. 6**B in Ref.[34] (*circles*) are superimposed. (*B*) Snapshots of numerical data; sheets 3 × 3 cm² simulating the RV (*top*) and LV (*bottom*). (*C*) Snapshots of numerical data in the combined RV-LV model of 6 × 6 cm². (*D*) DF map obtained from the model in panel *C*. Values in panels *B* and *C* are in milliseconds; in panel *D*, in Hertz. Broken lines in panels *C* and *D* show the perimeter of the LV model (area, 2 × 2 cm²). (*From* Samie FH, Mandapati R, Gray RA, et al. A mechanism of transition from ventricular fibrillation to tachycardia: effect of calcium channel blockade on the dynamics of rotating waves. Circ Res 2000;86:684–91; with permission.)

alpha-myosin heavy chain promoter.[44] Optical mapping of the epicardial surface of the ventricles showed that the Langendorff-perfused TG hearts were able to sustain stable VT/VF for almost 4 hours at an exceptionally high mean DF of about 45 Hz. In contrast, tachyarrhythmias in wild-type (WT) hearts lasted an average of ~3 seconds), and the mean DF was about 26 Hz. As shown in **Fig. 5**, volume-conducted ECGs, DF maps, and power spectral plots were obtained from representative WT and TG hearts in VF. In both cases the ECGs (top) are polymorphic and characteristic of VF, but the complexes are narrower in the TG compared with the WT heart. In the WT heart, the DF map (middle left) reveals a 33-Hz frequency domain (yellow) in addition to other slower domains, consistent with the power spectrum of the ECG trace (bottom left), which displays an extremely high DF of 34 Hz along with additional small peaks in an overall pattern that is typical of VF.[34,41] The DF map of the TG heart (middle right) shows a domain (white) of 56 Hz, coexisting with other slower frequency domains. The power

spectrum of the ECG (bottom right) has a large peak at 56 Hz coexisting with multiple other smaller peaks. Again, this pattern is indistinguishable from VF. Importantly, the stable, high-frequency, reentrant activity in both hearts slowed down, and eventually terminated in the presence of 10 μm Ba^{2+}, suggesting an important role for I_{K1}. Moreover, by increasing I_{K1} density in a two-dimensional computer model having realistic mouse ionic and action potential properties, a highly stable, fast rotor ($\approx$45 Hz) could be induced. Simulations suggested that the TG hearts allowed such a fast and stable rotor because of both greater outward I_{K1} conductance in cells at the core and shortened APD in the core vicinity, as well as increased excitability, in part because of faster recovery of Na^+ current.[41] The faster recovery of Na^+ current resulted in a larger rate of increase in the local conduction velocity as a function of the distance from the core in TG compared with WT hearts, in both simulations and experiments. In addition, simulations showed that rotor frequencies were more sensitive to

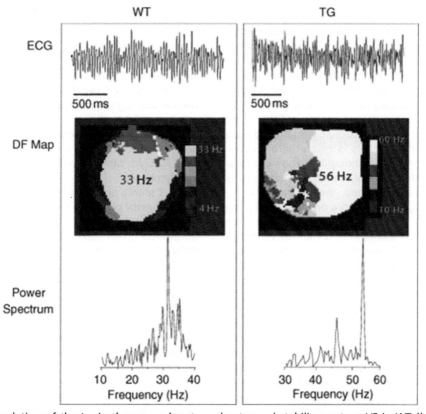

Fig. 5. Upregulation of the I_{K1} in the mouse heart accelerates and stabilizes rotors. VF in WT (*left*) and TG (*right*) hearts. (*Top*) ECGs (*middle*) DF maps, (*bottom*) corresponding power spectra of the ECG traces. Color scales: WT, 4 to 33 Hz; TG, 10 to 60 Hz. (*From* Noujaim SF, Pandit SV, Berenfeld O, et al. Up-regulation of the inward rectifier K+ current (I_{K1}) in the mouse heart accelerates and stabilizes rotors. J Physiol 2007;578:315–26; with permission.)

changes (doubling) in I_{K1}, compared with other K^+ currents.

MOLECULAR MECHANISMS THAT CONTROL VENTRICULAR FIBRILLATION FREQUENCY

Ventricular excitability is known to depend on the voltage-dependent properties of Kir2.1, which is mainly responsible for I_{K1}, and of the alpha subunit of the sodium channel $Na_V1.5$, which is responsible for I_{Na}. I_{K1} is the major current responsible for the maintenance of the resting membrane potential, whereas I_{Na} provides the largest fraction of the inward depolarizing current that flows during an action potential.[45] It is well known that a relationship between these two ionic currents is crucial for proper cardiac electrical function; disruption of this balance results in changes in sodium channel availability, cell excitability, APD, and conduction velocity.[46] Accordingly, I_{K1}-I_{Na} interactions are important in stabilizing and controlling the frequency of the electrical rotors that are responsible for the most dangerous cardiac arrhythmias, including VT and fibrillation.[47] Data in Kir2.1-overexpressing mice have provided strong evidence that the electrophysiologic interplay between I_{Na} and I_{K1} is essential in controlling the stability and frequency of reentry and VT/VF.[41] Moreover, as discussed earlier, I_{K1} upregulation is a substrate for very fast electrical rotors in structurally normal ventricles.

Recently, we provided strong evidence that the interplay between sodium and inward rectifier potassium channels is much more complex than was previously thought, involving mutual regulation at the protein level.[48] In single adult rat ventricular myocytes, we showed that I_{K1} increased significantly more on adenoviral transfer of Kir2.1 plus $Na_V1.5$ than when Kir2.1 was overexpressed alone; in neonatal rat ventricular myocyte (NRVM) monolayers, cooverexpression of $Na_V1.5$ with Kir2.1 increased conduction velocity, abbreviated APD, and increased rotor frequency beyond those produced by Kir2.1 overexpression alone; in TG mice overexpressing Kir2.1, peak I_{Na} density was twice as large as in the control; in heterozygous Kir2.1 knockout mice, $Na_V1.5$ protein was significantly reduced; and in human embryonic kidney cells $Na_V1.5$ overexpression induced retention of Kir2.1 in the membrane.[48] Further, preliminary data in mice showed that Scn5a reduction was accompanied by a concomitant reduction in I_{K1}. Importantly, our finding that coexpression of $Na_V1.5$ (with Kir2.1) may reduce internalization of Kir2.1 is a central mechanistic observation.[48]

Altogether, the evidence suggested that in cardiac cells there is model independent coregulation of Kir2.1 and $Na_V1.5$, which leads to the following question: what are the electrophysiologic consequences of the reciprocal regulation of $Na_V1.5$ and Kir2.1 on the frequency and dynamics of rotors?

To address this question and establish the role of cardiac excitability in the molecular control of VF frequency we used neonatal rat ventricular myocyte (NRVM) monolayers. Adenovirally mediated gene transfer enabled genetic manipulation through adenoviral gene transfer in a well-controlled environment in which stable two-dimensional rotors could be directly visualized.[48] First, we investigated the changes in the first derivative with respect to time of the action potential upstroke (dV/dt) and APD resulting from the molecular interplay between $Na_V1.5$ and Kir2.1 when 1 or both protein channels were overexpressed in isolated NRVMs. Current clamp recordings obtained from 4 different viral infection conditions showed that infection of a cell with Ad-$Na_V1.5$ alone hyperpolarized the resting membrane potential, increased the dV/dt, and prolonged the APD (**Fig. 6**). Infection with Ad-Kir2.1 alone also hyperpolarized the resting membrane potential and increased dV/dt. However, in this case, the APD was greatly abbreviated. In addition, in contrast with the effects of Ad-$Na_V1.5$ infection alone, infection with Ad-Kir2.1 plus $Na_V1.5$ resulted in a reproducible and significant reduction of the APD. The results predict that, because both excitability and APD are modified, genetic manipulation of ion channel expression in monolayers of electrically coupled cells should have important electrophysiologic consequences.

Fig. 7 shows phase maps (see **Fig. 7**A) and rotation frequency plots (see **Fig. 7**B) for NRVM monolayers infected with Ad-GFP (adenovirally transferred green fluorescent protein), Ad-$Na_V1.5$ alone, Ad-Kir2.1 alone, or a combination of Ad-$Na_V1.5$ plus Ad-Kir2.1. Color-coded signals in **Fig. 7**A indicate the phase in the excitation-recovery cycle at each pixel location.[41,49,50] Stable reentry was present in all monolayers, and in each there was a single stationary rotor. However, in single NRVMs, Ad-$Na_V1.5$ infection alone prolonged the APD (see **Fig. 6**). APD prolongation during reentry in the monolayer was manifest as a lengthening of the depolarization phases in the reentry cycle. Consequently, Ad-$Na_V1.5$ infection alone reduced the rotation frequency (see **Fig. 7**B). However, the shortened APD produced by Ad-Kir2.1 in neonatal cells (see **Fig. 6**) likely contributed to significantly decreased wavelength and increased rotation frequency (see **Fig. 7**). Most importantly, the

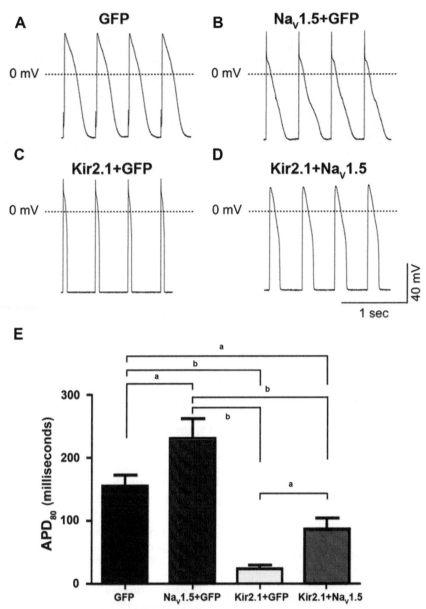

Fig. 6. $Na_V1.5$ and Kir2.1 cooverexpression significantly reduces the APD in single NRVMs paced at 2 Hz. (A–D) Action potential recordings from NRVMs infected with adenoviruses encoding (A) Green Fluorescent Protein (GFP) (n = 5); (B) $Na_V1.5$ plus GFP (n = 4); (C) Kir2.1 plus GFP (n = 4); (D) Kir2.1 plus $Na_V1.5$ (n = 5). (E) Summary plots of mean ± standard error of the mean APD_{80} for each group. Ad-GFP was used as an adenoviral control for single infections to account for the higher viral load expected as a result of Kir2.1 and $Na_V1.5$ coinfection (*red bar*). [a] *P*<.05; [b] *P*<.01. (*From* Milstein ML, Musa H, Balbuena DP, et al. Dynamic reciprocity of sodium and potassium channel expression in a macromolecular complex controls cardiac excitability and arrhythmia. Proc Natl Acad Sci U S A 2012;109:E2134–43; with permission.)

combined infection (Ad-$Na_V1.5$ plus Ad-Kir2.1) hyperpolarized the resting membrane potential, resulting in a shortened APD (see **Fig. 6**) and a faster conduction velocity.[48] Consequently, the frequency of reentry was even higher with cooverexpression of $Na_V1.5$ and Kir2.1 than Ad-Kir2.1 infection alone (see **Fig. 7B**). These results are also consistent with the idea of molecular interplay between $Na_V1.5$ and Kir2.1 channel proteins, and they also support that the underlying mechanism of this interplay is important in determining the frequency and stability of reentry in the normal heart.

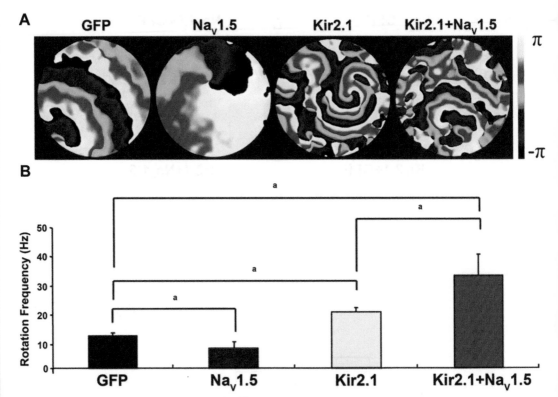

Fig. 7. Molecular Na$_V$1.5–Kir2.1 interactions modulate reentry frequency in NRVM monolayers. (*A*) Phase maps (3, 17, 18) for single rotations from representative optical mapping movies of monolayers infected with Ad-GFP, Ad-Na$_V$1.5, Ad-Kir2.1, or Ad-Kir2.1 plus Ad-Na$_V$1.5. The color bar indicates the phase in the excitation-recovery cycle. (*B*) Reentry frequencies in monolayers infected with Ad-GFP (*black*; n = 11), Ad-Na$_V$1.5 (*blue*; n = 13), Ad-Kir2.1 (*yellow*; n = 11), or Ad-Kir2.1 plus Ad-Na$_V$1.5 (*red*; n = 13). [a] $P<.01$ (analysis of variance). (*From* Milstein ML, Musa H, Balbuena DP, et al. Dynamic reciprocity of sodium and potassium channel expression in a macromolecular complex controls cardiac excitability and arrhythmia. Proc Natl Acad Sci U S A 2012;109:E2134–43; with permission.)

SUMMARY

Based on the data presented earlier, VF can no longer be considered to result from the random and aperiodic propagation of multiple independent wavelets throughout the cardiac muscle.[6] It also does not depend on the formation of a multi-spiral disordered state.[11] Careful application of concepts derived from the theory of nonlinear wave propagation to the problem of fibrillation in the heart and the advent of modern high-resolution mapping techniques, patch-clamping, and molecular biology and genetics has generated a new paradigm whereby the molecular, structural, and anatomic makeup of the ventricles support the self-organization of electrical waves into rotors that give rise to rapidly rotating spiral waves resulting in either predictable and organized monomorphic VT or more complex and turbulent patterns of VF, depending on the frequency of rotation and on the interaction of wave fronts with the cardiac muscle, both of which strongly depend on the molecular underpinnings of cardiac excitability, the spatial distribution of ion channels controlling excitability, and the anatomic structure of the ventricles. Cardiac diseases leading to changes in any such parameters should modify the behavior in what should be now predictable ways. As such, there is still hope for the development of a new generation of antifibrillatory agents that could, in the near future, be used as upstream prevention therapies for VF and make the intracardiac implantable defibrillator obsolete.

REFERENCES

1. Hayashi M, Shimizu W, Albert CM. The spectrum of epidemiology underlying sudden cardiac death. Circ Res 2015;116:1887–906.
2. Weisfeldt ML, Everson-Stewart S, Sitlani C, et al, Resuscitation Outcomes Consortium Investigators. Ventricular tachyarrhythmias after cardiac arrest in

public versus at home. N Engl J Med 2011;364: 313–21.

3. Jalife J, Gray RA, Morley GE, et al. Self-organization and the dynamical nature of ventricular fibrillation. Chaos 1998;8:79–93.

4. Jalife J. Ventricular fibrillation: mechanisms of initiation and maintenance. Annu Rev Physiol 2000;62: 25–50.

5. Wiggers C, Wiggers CJ. Studies of ventricular fibrillation caused by electric shock, ii: cinematographic and electrocardiographic observation of the natural process in the dog's heart. Its inhibition by potassium and the revival of coordinated beats by calcium. Am Heart J 1930;5:351–65.

6. Moe G. On the multiple wavelet hypothesis of atrial fibrillation. Arch Int Pharmacodyn Ther 1962;140: 183–8.

7. Winfree AT. Spiral waves of chemical activity. Science 1972;175:634–6.

8. Krinsky VI, Biktashev VN, Pertsov AM. Autowave approaches to cessation of reentrant arrhythmias. Ann N Y Acad Sci 1990;591:232–46.

9. Allessie MA, Bonke FIM, Schopman FJG. Circus movement in rabbit atrial muscle as a mechanism of tachycardia. III: the "leading circle" concept: a new model of circus movement in cardiac tissue without the involvement of an anatomical obstacle. Circ Res 1977;41:9–18.

10. Fenton FH, Cherry EM, Hastings HM, et al. Multiple mechanisms of spiral wave breakup in a model of cardiac electrical activity. Chaos 2002; 12:852–92.

11. Karma A. Electrical alternans and spiral wave breakup in cardiac tissue. Chaos 1994;4:461–72.

12. Riccio ML, Koller ML, Gilmour RF Jr. Electrical restitution and spatiotemporal organization during ventricular fibrillation. Circ Res 1999;84:955–63.

13. Chen PS, Wolf PD, Dixon EG, et al. Mechanism of ventricular vulnerability to single premature stimuli in open-chest dogs. Circ Res 1988;62:1191–209.

14. Witkowski FX, Leon LJ, Penkoske PA, et al. Spatiotemporal evolution of ventricular fibrillation. Nature 1998;392:78–82.

15. Fenton FH, Cherry EM, Karma A, et al. Modeling wave propagation in realistic heart geometries using the phase-field method. Chaos 2005;15:013502.

16. Weiss JN, Garfinkel A, Karagueuzian HS, et al. Chaos and the transition to ventricular fibrillation: a new approach to antiarrhythmic drug evaluation. Circulation 1999;99:2819–26.

17. Nolasco JB, Dahlen RW. A graphic method for the study of alternation in cardiac action potentials. J Appl Physiol 1968;25:191–6.

18. Chialvo DR, Gilmour RF Jr, Jalife J. Low dimensional chaos in cardiac tissue. Nature 1990;343:653–7.

19. Watanabe M, Otani NF, Gilmour RF Jr. Biphasic restitution of action potential duration and complex dynamics in ventricular myocardium. Circ Res 1995;76:915–21.

20. Gilmour RF Jr, Otani NF, Watanabe MA. Memory and complex dynamics in cardiac Purkinje fibers. Am J Physiol 1997;272:H1826–32.

21. Fenton F, Karma A. Vortex dynamics in three-dimensional continuous myocardium with fiber rotation: filament instability and fibrillation. Chaos 1998; 8:20–47.

22. Davidenko JM, Pertsov AV, Salomonsz R, et al. Stationary and drifting spiral waves of excitation in isolated cardiac muscle. Nature 1992;355:349–51.

23. Pertsov AM, Davidenko JM, Salomonsz R, et al. Spiral waves of excitation underlie reentrant activity in isolated cardiac muscle. Circ Res 1993; 72:631–50.

24. Gray RA, Jalife J, Panfilov AV, et al. Mechanisms of cardiac fibrillation. Science 1995;270:1222–3 [author reply: 1224–5].

25. Gray RA, Pertsov AM, Jalife J. Spatial and temporal organization during cardiac fibrillation. Nature 1998; 392:75–8.

26. Jalife J. Deja vu in the theories of atrial fibrillation dynamics. Cardiovasc Res 2011;89:766–75.

27. Samie FH, Mandapati R, Gray RA, et al. A mechanism of transition from ventricular fibrillation to tachycardia: effect of calcium channel blockade on the dynamics of rotating waves. Circ Res 2000; 86:684–91.

28. Jalife J, Berenfeld O, Mansour M. Mother rotors and fibrillatory conduction: a mechanism of atrial fibrillation. Cardiovasc Res 2002;54:204–16.

29. Jalife J, Berenfeld O, Skanes A, et al. Mechanisms of atrial fibrillation: mother rotors or multiple daughter wavelets, or both? J Cardiovasc Electrophysiol 1998;9:S2–12.

30. Chen J, Mandapati R, Berenfeld O, et al. Dynamics of wavelets and their role in atrial fibrillation in the isolated sheep heart. Cardiovasc Radiol 2000;48: 220–32.

31. Zaitsev AV, Berenfeld O, Mironov SF, et al. Distribution of excitation frequencies on the epicardial and endocardial surfaces of fibrillating ventricular wall of the sheep heart. Circ Res 2000;86:408–17.

32. Schmidt-Nielsen K. Scaling: why is animal size so important? Cambridge (United Kingdom): Cambridge University Press; 1984.

33. Noujaim SF, Berenfeld O, Kalifa J, et al. Universal scaling law of electrical turbulence in the mammalian heart. Proc Natl Acad Sci U S A 2007;104: 20985–9.

34. Samie FH, Berenfeld O, Anumonwo J, et al. Rectification of the background potassium current: a determinant of rotor dynamics in ventricular fibrillation. Circ Res 2001;89:1216–23.

35. Gray RA, Jalife J, Panfilov A, et al. Nonstationary vortexlike reentrant activity as a mechanism of

polymorphic ventricular tachycardia in the isolated rabbit heart. Circulation 1995;91:2454–69.

36. Boersma L, Brugada J, Kirchhof C, et al. Mapping of reset of anatomic and functional reentry in aniso-tropic rabbit ventricular myocardium. Circulation 1994;89:852–62.

37. Priori SG, Napolitano C, Cantu F, et al. Differential response to Na+ channel blockade, β-adrenergic stimulation, and rapid pacing in a cellular model mimicking the SCN5A and HERG defects present in the long-QT syndrome. Circ Res 1996; 78:1009–15.

38. Beaumont J, Davidenko N, Davidenko JM, et al. Spi-ral waves in two-dimensional models of ventricular muscle: formation of a stationary core. Biophys J 1998;75:1–14.

39. Beaumont J, Jalife J. Rotors and spiral waves in two dimensions. In: Zipes DP, Jalife J, editors. Cardiac electrophysiology from cell to bedside. Saunders; 2000. p. 327–35.

40. Miake J, Marban E, Nuss HB. Functional role of in-ward rectifier current in heart probed by kir2.1 over-expression and dominant-negative suppression. J Clin Invest 2003;111:1529–36.

41. Noujaim SF, Pandit SV, Berenfeld O, et al. Up-regulation of the inward rectifier K+ current (IK1) in the mouse heart accelerates and stabilizes rotors. J Physiol 2007;578:315–26.

42. Deo M, Ruan Y, Pandit SV, et al. Kcnj2 mutation in short QT syndrome 3 results in atrial fibrillation and ventricular proarrhythmia. Proc Natl Acad Sci U S A 2013;110:4291–6.

43. Warren M, Guha PK, Berenfeld O, et al. Blockade of the inward rectifying potassium current terminates ventricular fibrillation in the guinea pig heart. J Cardiovasc Electrophysiol 2003;14:621–31.

44. Li J, McLerie M, Lopatin AN. Transgenic up-regulation of IK1 in the mouse heart leads to multiple abnormalities of cardiac excitability. Am J Physiol Heart Circ Physiol 2004;287(6):H2790–802.

45. Fozzard HA, Hanck DA. Structure and function of voltage-dependent sodium channels: comparison of brain II and cardiac isoforms. Physiol Rev 1996; 76:887–926.

46. Lopatin AN, Nichols CG. Inward rectifiers in the heart: an update on I(K1). J Mol Cell Cardiol 2001; 33:625–38.

47. Noujaim SF, Auerbach DS, Jalife J. Ventricular fibril-lation: dynamics and ion channel determinants. Circ J 2007;71(Suppl A):A1–11.

48. Milstein ML, Musa H, Balbuena DP, et al. Dynamic reciprocity of sodium and potassium channel expression in a macromolecular complex controls cardiac excitability and arrhythmia. Proc Natl Acad Sci U S A 2012;109:E2134–43.

49. Cerrone M, Noujaim SF, Tolkacheva EG, et al. Arrhythmogenic mechanisms in a mouse model of catecholaminergic polymorphic ventricular tachy-cardia. Circ Res 2007;101:1039–48.

50. Munoz V, Grzeda KR, Desplantez T, et al. Adeno-viral expression of IKs contributes to wavebreak and fibrillatory conduction in neonatal rat ventricu-lar cardiomyocyte monolayers. Circ Res 2007; 101:475–83.

Ventricular Arrhythmias in Apparently Normal Hearts
Who Needs an Implantable Cardiac Defibrillator?

Alex Y. Tan, MD[a,b,*], Kenneth Ellenbogen, MD, FHRS[b]

KEYWORDS

- Implantable cardiac defibrillator • Ventricular arrhythmia • Sudden cardiac arrest
- Premature ventricular complex

KEY POINTS

- Ventricular arrhythmias in patients without apparent heart disease are mostly benign; however, a small subset of patients may develop malignant ventricular arrhythmias, including monomorphic ventricular tachycardia (VT), polymorphic VT, and ventricular fibrillation (VF).
- The initiating malignant premature ventricular complex (PVC) often arises from locations similar to benign PVCs. The mechanisms by which otherwise benign PVCs trigger malignant sustained arrhythmias are not fully elucidated; therefore, therapies run the full gamut of the electrophysiologic spectrum, including radiofrequency ablation, antiarrhythmic medications, and implantable cardiac defibrillators (ICDs).
- ICDs are indicated for patients who survived VF arrest. ICDs should be considered for patients with high-risk features, such as syncope, and have nonsustained VT with malignant electrocardiographic criteria on Holter or telemetry.
- Where uncertainty exists, a thorough workup is necessary to elucidate the long-term arrhythmic prognosis, which includes MRI, ambulatory rhythm monitoring, and longitudinal clinical follow-up including periodic repetition of the aforementioned workup.
- In addition to a reversible cardiomyopathy, frequent PVCs may also induce a distinct form of cellular electrophysiologic remodeling characterized by increased action potential duration and cellular repolarization heterogeneity, an electrical substrate that may promote reentrant ventricular arrhythmias.

INTRODUCTION

Implantable cardiac defibrillators (ICDs) are the mainstay of therapy for patients with cardiomyopathy (CM) who are at high risk for malignant ventricular arrhythmias and consequently sudden cardiac death.[1] The benefits of ICDs in this group have been well documented in large clinical trials.[2–7] However, patients without apparent structural heart disease, or those with mildly impaired left ventricular ejection fraction (LVEF 40-50%), constitute most (>80%) patients who

[a] Electrophysiology Section, Division of Cardiology, Hunter Holmes McGuire VA Medical Center, 1201 Broad Rock Boulevard, Richmond, VA 23249, USA; [b] VCU Pauley Heart Center, Medical College of Virginia, Virginia Commonwealth University School of Medicine, 1250 E Marshall Street, Richmond, VA 23298, USA
* Corresponding author. Hunter Holmes McGuire VA Medical Center, 1201 Broad Rock Boulevard, Richmond, VA 23249.
E-mail address: alex.tan@va.gov

Card Electrophysiol Clin 8 (2016) 613–621
http://dx.doi.org/10.1016/j.ccep.2016.04.010
1877-9182/16/$ – see front matter Published by Elsevier Inc.

experience sudden cardiac death.[8,9] These patients are not well represented in clinical trials[2–6] and belong to a heterogeneous group whereby the individual benefits of ICD therapy are less clear-cut. Patients with idiopathic ventricular arrhythmias (IVA) fall into this category. By definition, IVA occurs in the absence of known structural heart disease detected by conventional imaging and, in most cases, by a nonreentrant arrhythmia mechanism with foci from certain locations, such as the ventricular outflow tract region, aortic cusps, His-Purkinje conduction system, atrioventricular valvular annuli, or papillary muscles.[10–13] These patients typically present with premature ventricular complexes (PVCs) or nonsustained ventricular tachycardia (NSVT). Thus, this is essentially a very large and heterogeneous group of different patient types. Within this group is a small subset of patients who may experience malignant ventricular arrhythmias in the form of monomorphic (MM) VT, polymorphic (PM) VT, or ventricular fibrillation (VF).[14] More recently, frequent PVCs (>20% burden) have been recognized to induce a potentially reversible form of CM with a prevalence of systolic dysfunction as high as 50% in patients presenting for PVC ablation.[15–17] Patients with a malignant arrhythmic presentation, or those with incompletely reversible systolic dysfunction due to a variety of reasons, are 2 groups of patients who are potential candidates for ICD therapy. Note that there are 2 other groups of patients without LV systolic dysfunction who might be prone to malignant ventricular arrhythmias and be ICD candidates, namely, those with inherited channelopathies, such as congenital long QT syndrome or Brugada syndrome, and those with specific structural derangements, such as hypertrophic CM and arrhythmogenic right ventricular dysplasia. However, ICD indications in these groups are outside the focus of this article.

PREVALENCE OF MALIGNANT VENTRICULAR ARRHYTHMIAS AND POTENTIAL IMPLANTABLE CARDIAC DEFIBRILLATOR BURDEN

To determine the potential burden of ICD therapy in this group, it is useful to examine the prevalence of malignant arrhythmias in patients with IVA. A survey of the literature, however, quickly reveals an absence of robust epidemiologic data to support any major conclusions. Sudden cardiac death was first reported in 1975 in a young patient with right ventricular outflow tract (RVOT) PVCs whose only prior symptom was palpitations.[18] Since then, most reported cases of idiopathic PVC-induced VF and sudden cardiac death have been in

Purkinje-related VF.[15] Several case series have examined RVOT PVC-triggered malignant ventricular arrhythmias[14,15,17,19] and reported a prevalence of between 7% and 16% of malignant RVOT arrhythmias among a small group of patients presenting with RVOT PVC ablation. For example, Noda and colleagues[14] reported that 16 patients out of 101 consecutive patients (16%) who presented for ablation of RVOT PVCs had initiation of PM VT (N = 11) and VF (N = 5) by RVOT PVCs. In 2 other studies,[15,20] the investigators studied patients who had spontaneous VF or PM VT and found that 1 out of 14 patients (7%)[20] and 4 out of 27 (15%) patients had initiating PVCs arising from an RVOT origin.[15] The actual prevalence of malignant ventricular arrhythmias in patients with IVA is likely to be lower due to inherent referral bias and small numbers in these studies. The prevalence of malignant arrhythmias triggered by IVA from other foci[10,21] remains unclear.

PROPOSED MECHANISM FOR MALIGNANT ARRHYTHMIAS

The mechanisms of malignant arrhythmias have important implications to discriminate the need for long-term ICD therapy. A key feature to distinguish malignant arrhythmias triggered by IVA from idiopathic VF is to identify the triggering PVC as being unifocal (unlike, for example, fascicular VT or VF, which may be reentrant) and identical in origin to putatively benign PVCs that coexist in the same patient. The question is what leads to conversion of otherwise benign PVCs to malignant sustained arrhythmias?

The outflow tract artery junction is complex both in terms of its development and histology with multiple tissue types interfacing in this region.[22] Myocardial sleeves extend into the great arteries for variable distances and commonly extend into each of the 3 pulmonary valve cusps and beyond by up to 2 cm into the PA, analogous to the relationship between pulmonary vein and left atrium.[22,23] This anisotropy in the absence of organic conduction disease supports the hypothesis of slow conduction or functional conduction block of a rapid-firing focus leading to chaotic degeneration to PM VT or VF.[19,24] Rapid burst pacing from the origin of the VT can reproduce PM QRS, lending further support to the theory of delayed conduction in the vicinity of a PVC focus (Fig. 1).[14,19,24] Alternatively, localized anisotropy promotes microreentry from a single PVC focus, with subsequent degeneration to fast VT or VF. Third, multiple firing foci may be present given that the outflow tract region can contain remnants

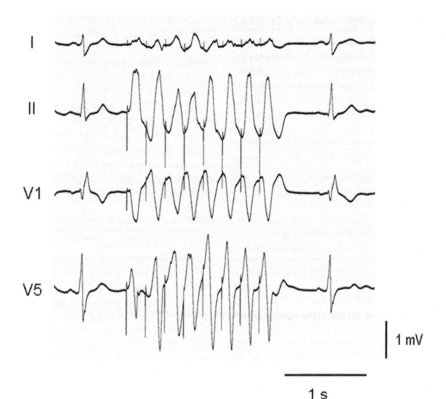

Fig. 1. PM changes of the QRS complex on electrocardiographic leads I, II, V1, and V5 during rapid pacing in a patient with the malignant form of idiopathic VT originating from RVOT. The morphologic changes were induced by rapid pacing from the origin of the initiating VPC, which was confirmed by the efficacy of radiofrequency catheter ablation. VPC, ventricular premature complex. (*From* Noda T, Shimizu W, Taguchi A, et al. Malignant entity of idiopathic ventricular fibrillation and polymorphic ventricular tachycardia initiated by premature extrasystoles originating from the right ventricular outflow tract. J Am Coll Cardiol 2005;46(7):1292; with permission.)

of embryonic cardiac tissue that continue to exhibit nodelike spontaneous depolarizations.[25,26] Under certain conditions, such as catecholamine excess, multiple firing foci may lead to the appearance of PM QRS. Ablation of the single firing focus eliminates the source of triggered activity, and adjacent ablations may eliminate nearby triggers and modify the substrate for slowed conduction.[15,24]

RISK FACTORS FOR MALIGNANT VENTRICULAR ARRHYTHMIAS

In general, patients with IVA who present with malignant symptoms (cardiac arrest or syncope) are considered to possess an electrical substrate that portends a higher recurrence of malignant arrhythmias than those who do not.[14,15,17] In addition, several key electrocardiographic (ECG) predictors of risk have emerged based on small retrospective case series. **Box 1** summarizes the high-risk ECG and clinical features of malignant PVCs.[14,15,17,19] In general, malignant features include (1) shorter coupled initiating or second

PVC beat, either of which may decrease on the vulnerable portion of the T wave; (2) shorter cycle length (CL) of malignant VT than benign VT; (3) longer QRS duration; and (4) disorganized morphology reflecting abnormal conduction and abnormal electrical substrate.

Box 1
Summary of high-risk features of malignant ventricular arrhythmias

ECG Features

- Short coupling interval of first or second PVC beat
- Short cycle length of NSVT
- Longer QRS duration
- Morphology: VF > PM VT > MM VT

Symptoms

- Cardiac arrest
- History of syncope

History of Aborted Sudden Death or Syncope

Noda and colleagues[14] reported that a previous history of syncope with malignant characteristics was more frequently observed in the 7 patients with malignant RVOT VT than in 85 patients with benign RVOT VT (5 of 7 vs 15 of 85; $P = .005$). Thus, a history of syncope with malignant characteristics may be a predictor of the coexistence of malignant VF or PM VT in patients with idiopathic VT originating from RVOT. Unfortunately, the absence of symptoms may not necessarily be reassuring because many patients with VF arrest had only benign palpitations previously.[17,24]

Shorter Coupling Interval of the First or Second Premature Ventricular Complex Beat

The coupling interval (CI) of the first PVC beat that initiates VT or VF is often[17] but not always shorter[14,19] than isolated benign outflow tract PVCs and may decrease on the vulnerable portion of the T wave to induce fast MM VT, PM VT, or VF. Viskin and colleagues[17] found that the first PVC beat (300 ±40 ms) that initiated idiopathic VF (Purkinje derived) was shorter than that which induced malignant RVOT VT (340 ± 30 ms); however, the latter was in turn shorter than that of benign RVOT VT (427 ± 76 ms). Noda and colleagues[14] made similar observations, but the difference between malignant RVOT VT versus benign RVOT VT (409 ± 62 vs 428 ± 65 ms) did not meet statistical significance. When the CI of the first beat was comparable, Kim and colleagues[27] found that the CI of the second beat of NSVT was significantly shorter in the malignant compared with the benign group (313 ± 58 ms vs 385 ± 83 ms, $P<.01$). Thus, these data underscore the fact that shorter coupled PVCs are a risk factor for triggering of malignant VA; however, a definite cut-off between benign and malignant remains elusive. Second, absolute CIs that initiate malignant arrhythmias may be site specific, with the aforementioned data derived exclusively from RVOT PVCs. For example, Purkinje PVCs that initiate idiopathic VF tend to have shorter CIs than those of RVOT initiating VF (355 ± 30 vs 280 ± 26 ms; $P = .01$).[15] Third, a longer CI does not necessarily imply an absence of risk, as it is conceivable that both short and long CIs may coexist in the same patients who have both benign and malignant PVCs. Unfortunately, in the aforementioned studies, those internal comparisons were not made.

Shorter CL

A faster CL of arrhythmia may be associated with greater likelihood of fibrillatory degeneration.

Noda and colleagues[14] found that malignant PM VT (N = 17) had a shorter CL than benign forms of MM RVOT VT (N = 85) (245 ± 28 vs 328 ± 65 ms; $P = .0001$). When benign MM VT and malignant PM VT were present in the same patients (**Fig. 2**), the CL of malignant PM VT (see **Fig. 2**B) was significantly shorter than benign MM VT (see **Fig. 2**A) (273 ± 23 vs 241 ± 36 ms; N = 7, $P = .08$), which in turn was shorter than benign MM VT in other patients without malignant arrhythmias (N = 85, 273 ± 23 vs 328 ± 65 ms; $P = .0001$).

QRS Duration of Ventricular Tachycardia

Noda and colleagues[14] reported a significantly longer QRS duration of malignant versus benign RVOT VT (148 ± 8 vs 142 ± 12 ms). A longer QRS duration of the VT (and/or sinus rhythm) may reflect the presence of intrinsic electrical disease and slowed conduction that may promote conversion of benign PVCs to PM VT or VF.

Prematurity Index

Igarashi and colleagues[28] suggested that a prematurity index (CI of PVC/sinus cycle length) of 0.73 or less distinguishes malignant from benign PVCs with a sensitivity of 91% and specificity of 44%. However, this has not been validated.

Disorganized Morphology

Most symptomatic malignant arrhythmias are disorganized and associated more commonly with PM VT or VF than MM VT.[15,17,19,24] PM QRS may reflect the presence of more than one focus of arrhythmia[27] or derive from a single focus with anisotropic conduction or localized microreentry in the vicinity.

CANDIDATES FOR IMPLANTABLE CARDIAC DEFIBRILLATOR THERAPY

The authors present 4 scenarios in which ICDs are considered and discuss the rationale for their suggested approach in each case.

Survivors of Cardiac Arrest: Implantable Cardiac Defibrillator or Ablation?

Despite uncertainties in the mechanisms and risk stratification of sudden cardiac death, there is general consensus that ICDs are indicated in survivors of cardiac arrest due to VF, even if the initiating PVC can be mapped and successfully ablated. Radiofrequency (RF) ablation can

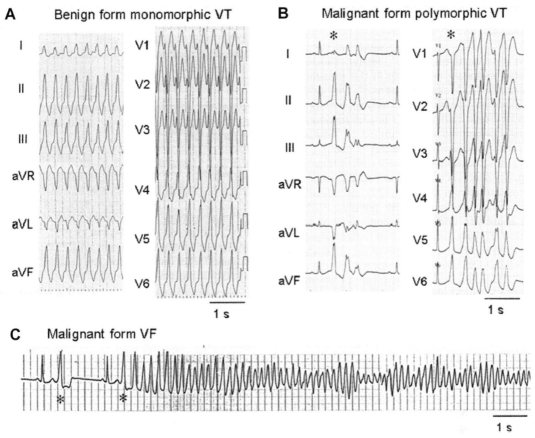

Fig. 2. Malignant MM (*A*), PM VT (*B*), and VF (*C*) from the same patient. Note that the initiating PVC (*) is identical in all cases, with a left bundle branch block inferior axis late precordial transition morphology consistent with RVOT. (*From* Noda T, Shimizu W, Taguchi A, et al. Malignant entity of idiopathic ventricular fibrillation and polymorphic ventricular tachycardia initiated by premature extrasystoles originating from the right ventricular outflow tract. J Am Coll Cardiol 2005;46(7):1289; with permission.)

eliminate idiopathic outflow tract PVCs[11] and PVC triggers for VF from RVOT and Purkinje network[15] with an 80% to 90% success rate resulting in no recurrent VF or sudden death after 2 years despite limited recurrence of PVCs.[15] Thus, it might be tempting to assume that ablation can cure malignant arrhythmias, eliminate the risk of sudden cardiac death, and obviate an ICD. Moreover, Viskin and colleagues[17] reported 3 patients with the malignant form of idiopathic RVOT VT treated with ablation in one patient and ICD implantation in the remaining 2 patients, with all 3 free of arrhythmia between 2 and 8 years of follow-up despite 2 patients with ICDs not receiving any ablation therapy. Noda and colleagues[14] performed ablation in 16 patients with the malignant form of idiopathic VT arising from RVOT with an ICD was implanted in one patient with induced VF after ablation and beta-blockers in 4 others with partial ablation success.

They found no recurrence of syncope, VF, or cardiac arrest after 2 years. Thus, in spite of a malignant initial presentation, the long-term outlook in the absence of structural heart disease may be more benign than in structural heart disease. Nevertheless, there are some isolated case reports of a late malignant recurrence of arrhythmia in spite of successful ablation.[29,30] Second, the difficulty with an ablation-only approach lies in identifying the precise PVC trigger to ablate and the lack of long-term outcomes data following ablation. Third, even if focal ablation can eliminate the trigger, it is unclear if it can fully eliminate the more regional or globally distributed electrical substrate that promotes fibrillatory degeneration. Fourth, some types of PVCs have a higher recurrence rate, particularly papillary muscle, intramural, and septal PVCs; others, such as Purkinje PVCs, can develop new ones in other parts of the network.

History of Syncope and Nonsustained Ventricular Tachycardia

If there was a history of suspicious syncope, then nonsustained VT on Holter should be treated seriously, especially in the presence of malignant ECG characteristics.[19] The value of an Electrophysiologic (EP) study as a diagnostic and risk stratification tool remains unclear; it is usually performed in the context of therapeutic ablation. However, an EP study is useful if it reproduces sustained VT/VF with provocation (**Fig. 3**), identifies the precise PVC trigger of sustained arrhythmia (see **Fig. 2C**), or reproduces with rapid pacing from the putative PVC site the same PM QRS morphology as that of the clinical VT (see **Fig. 3**). In this perfect combination of a malignant outcome of an EP study, an ICD should be strongly considered. On the other hand, the absence of inducible VT/VF in the context of suspicious syncope may not necessarily be reassuring because the yield of provocative studies is generally low. The influence of a successful ablation outcome on decisions regarding ICDs in this cohort also remains an unsettled issue.

Asymptomatic with Nonsustained Ventricular Tachycardia with Malignant Electrocardiogram Criteria

In the absence of any symptoms (no syncope, presyncope, or cardiac arrest), it is unclear if NSVT even in the presence of malignant ECG characteristics (fast NSVT, short CI of first or second PVC beat, wide QRS duration of PVCs) is sufficient to warrant ICD therapy. Close longitudinal follow-up with repeat Holter/event monitor, EP study, and MRI to rule out late development of scarring may be helpful to aid this decision.

Premature Ventricular Complex–Induced Cardiomyopathy and Implantable Cardiac Defibrillators

Frequent PVCs can induce LV systolic dysfunction, which is reversible with successful ablation of PVCs.[11,31,32] In a canine model, PVC-induced CM is characterized by the absence of fibrosis and inflammation,[16] unlike other forms of systolic CM.[33] Therefore, the presence of PVC-induced CM per se should not warrant an ICD. However, frequent PVCs can also induce cellular electrophysiologic remodeling in the form of downregulation of outward potassium current IK_s, leading to increased action potential duration and repolarization heterogeneity.[34] Abnormal repolarization heterogeneity may promote reentrant ventricular arrhythmias. Action potential prolongation also promotes early after depolarization-mediated triggered activity.[35,36] Thus, beyond the mechanical dysfunction caused by frequent PVCs, cellular electrical remodeling may be proarrhythmic. Because this remodeling is distinct from other types of systolic cardiomyopathy,[34] the mechanism of remodeling is likely the result of a PVC syndrome rather than a nonspecific manifestation of a heart failure. Thus, it is possible that the elimination of PVCs will result in resolution of cellular remodeling in parallel with the recovery of

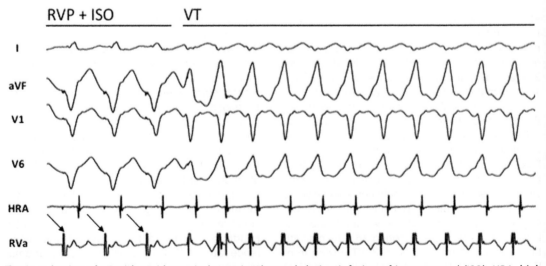

Fig. 3. Induction of VT with rapid ventricular pacing (*arrows*) during infusion of isoproterenol (ISO). HRA, high right atrium; Rva, right ventricular apex; RVP, right ventricular pacing. (*Adapted from* Lerman BB. Outflow tract ventricular arrhythmias: an update. Trends Cardiovasc Med 2015;25(6):556; with permission.)

systolic function,[16] though this remains unproven. Therefore, the concurrent presence of high PVC burden, PVC-induced CM, and malignant arrhythmic presentations may represent a heightened state of proarrhythmia, in which case wearable defibrillator therapy is recommended until LVEF recovers.

Influence of a Mixed Substrate on Implantable Cardiac Defibrillator Therapy

IVAs by definition occur in patients without apparent structural heart disease. However, they are also common in patients with structural heart disease in which the arrhythmias have a nonreentrant mechanism unrelated to scarring. In one series of 97 patients with IVA presenting for ablation, 43% of patients had preexisting structural heart disease.[37] Patients with preexisting mild systolic dysfunction might develop a superimposed PVC-induced CM resulting in deterioration of LVEF to an extent whereby they meet criteria for primary prevention ICD implantation.[1] In addition to IVA unrelated to the underlying cardiac substrate, patients with structural heart disease are also more likely to have left-sided and multifocal PVCs related to scar and less amenable to RF ablation.[37,38] Therefore, recovery of LVEF in the case of a superimposed PVC-induced CM is more likely to be incomplete.[38] These data may have significant implications for ICD therapy. The optimal approach to permanent ICD implantation remains unrefined and needs to be individualized, however, wearable defibrillator therapy should be considered in high-risk individuals while awaiting improvement in LVEF following catheter ablation or pharmacologic suppression.

SUGGESTED APPROACH TO IMPLANTABLE CARDIAC DEFIBRILLATOR RISK STRATIFICATION

Most patients with IVA have a benign prognosis and will not require an ICD. However, in a subset of patients with malignant symptoms or arrhythmias with ECG criteria, clarifying the risk of sudden cardiac death is an important first step to determine the need for an ICD. At present no single criterion accurately identifies patients who may be at risk of sudden cardiac death from VT/VF. The authors' suggested approach (**Fig. 4**) includes

1. Obtain a comprehensive history to tease out any evidence of prior syncope.
2. Conduct an MRI to rule out structural abnormalities,[39,40] in particular of arrhythmogenic right ventricular CM in the case of RVOT PVCs.
3. Use an event monitor or implantable loop recorder to document the presence of spontaneous episodes of VT that may have malignant ECG characterisitics.[19]
4. Consider provocative EP study to induce arrhythmia and identify PVC trigger.
5. Because of the infrequency of events, longitudinal clinical follow-up with repetition of the aforementioned studies may be needed, as structural abnormalities may become apparent over time[19] and initial benign presentation

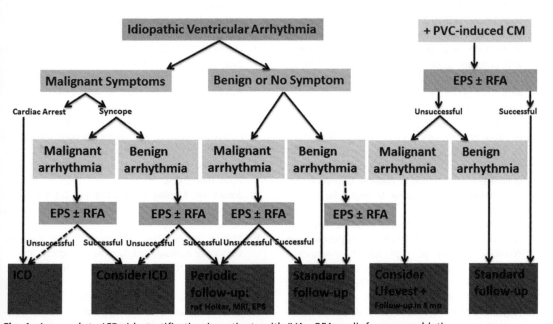

Fig. 4. Approach to ICD risk stratification in patients with IVAs. RFA, radiofrequency ablation.

may not reassure against a malignant outcome later.[15]

Ultimately, we need better long-term follow-up data from patient registries or multicenter studies in order to better discriminate patients at high risk for malignant arrhythmias.

SUMMARY

A small subset of patients with IVAs without apparent heart disease may experience malignant ventricular arrhythmias, such as rapid MM VT, PM VT, or VF. The predictors of a malignant arrhythmic presentation remain unsettled. Although the PVC triggers for malignant arrhythmias can be successfully ablated with a high success rate, long-term outcomes following ablation are unknown. ICDs are indicated for survivors of cardiac arrest. As more data become available on other high-risk patient subsets, such as those with syncope and nonsustained VT with malignant ECG features, or those with PVC-induced CM with incomplete recovery, the indications for ICDs will likely evolve as our understanding of their long-term arrhythmic risk improves.

REFERENCES

1. Kusumoto FM, Calkins H, Boehmer J, et al. HRS/ACC/AHA expert consensus statement on the use of implantable cardioverter-defibrillator therapy in patients who are not included or not well represented in clinical trials. Circulation 2014;130:94–125.

2. Bardy GH, Lee KL, Mark DB, et al. Amiodarone or an implantable cardioverter-defibrillator for congestive heart failure. N Engl J Med 2005;352(3):225–37.

3. Buxton AE, Lee KL, Fisher JD, et al. A randomized study of the prevention of sudden death in patients with coronary artery disease. Multicenter Unsustained Tachycardia Trial Investigators. N Engl J Med 1999;341(25):1882–90.

4. Hohnloser SH, Kuck K-H, Dorian P, et al. Prophylactic use of an implantable cardioverter-defibrillator after acute myocardial infarction. N Engl J Med 2004; 351(24):2481–8.

5. Kadish A, Dyer A, Daubert JP, et al. Prophylactic defibrillator implantation in patients with nonischemic dilated cardiomyopathy. N Engl J Med 2004; 350(21):2151–8.

6. Moss AJ, Hall WJ, Cannom DS, et al. Improved survival with an implanted defibrillator in patients with coronary disease at high risk for ventricular arrhythmia. Multicenter Automatic Defibrillator Implantation Trial Investigators. N Engl J Med 1996;335(26):1933–40.

7. Nogami A, Naito S, Tada H, et al. Verapamil-sensitive left anterior fascicular ventricular tachycardia: results of radiofrequency ablation in six patients. J Cardiovasc Electrophysiol 1998;9(12):1269–78.

8. Myerburg RJ, Kessler KM, Castellanos A. Sudden cardiac death: epidemiology, transient risk, and intervention assessment. Ann Intern Med 1993; 119(12):1187–97.

9. Wellens HJJ, Schwartz PJ, Lindemans FW, et al. Risk stratification for sudden cardiac death: current status and challenges for the future. Eur Heart J 2014;35(25):1642–51.

10. Al'Aref SJ, Ip JE, Markowitz SM, et al. Differentiation of papillary muscle from fascicular and mitral annular ventricular arrhythmias in patients with and without structural heart disease. Circ Arrhythm Electrophysiol 2015;8(3):616–24.

11. Bogun F, Crawford T, Reich S, et al. Radiofrequency ablation of frequent, idiopathic premature ventricular complexes: comparison with a control group without intervention. Heart Rhythm 2007;4(7):863–7.

12. Kawamura M, Hsu JC, Vedantham V, et al. Clinical and electrocardiographic characteristics of idiopathic ventricular arrhythmias with right bundle branch block and superior axis: comparison of apical crux area and posterior septal left ventricle. Heart Rhythm 2015;12(6):1137–44.

13. Lerman BB, Stein K, Engelstein ED, et al. Mechanism of repetitive monomorphic ventricular tachycardia. Circulation 1995;92(3):421–9.

14. Noda T, Shimizu W, Taguchi A, et al. Malignant entity of idiopathic ventricular fibrillation and polymorphic ventricular tachycardia initiated by premature extrasystoles originating from the right ventricular outflow tract. J Am Coll Cardiol 2005; 46(7):1288–94.

15. Haïssaguerre M, Shoda M, Jaïs P, et al. Mapping and ablation of idiopathic ventricular fibrillation. Circulation 2002;106(8):962–7.

16. Huizar JF, Kaszala K, Potfay J, et al. Left ventricular systolic dysfunction induced by ventricular ectopy: a novel model for premature ventricular contraction-induced cardiomyopathy. Circ Arrhythm Electrophysiol 2011;4(4):543–9.

17. Viskin S, Rosso R, Rogowski O, et al. The "short-coupled" variant of right ventricular outflow ventricular tachycardia: a not-so-benign form of benign ventricular tachycardia? J Cardiovasc Electrophysiol 2005;16(8):912–6.

18. James TN, Marilley RJ, Marriott HJ. De subitaneis mortibus. XI. Young girl with palpitations. Circulation 1975;51(4):743–8.

19. Shimizu W. Arrhythmias originating from the right ventricular outflow tract: how to distinguish "malignant" from "benign"? Heart Rhythm 2009;6(10): 1507–11.

20. Leenhardt A, Glaser E, Burguera M, et al. Short-coupled variant of torsade de pointes. A new electrocardiographic entity in the spectrum of idiopathic

ventricular tachyarrhythmias. Circulation 1994;89(1):206–15.

21. Kawamura M, Gerstenfeld EP, Vedantham V, et al. Idiopathic ventricular arrhythmia originating from the cardiac crux or inferior septum: epicardial idiopathic ventricular arrhythmia. Circ Arrhythm Electrophysiol 2014;7(6):1152–8.

22. Asirvatham SJ. Correlative anatomy for the invasive electrophysiologist: outflow tract and supravalvar arrhythmia. J Cardiovasc Electrophysiol 2009;20(8):955–68.

23. Liu CF, Cheung JW, Thomas G, et al. Ubiquitous myocardial extensions into the pulmonary artery demonstrated by integrated intracardiac echocardiography and electroanatomic mapping: changing the paradigm of idiopathic right ventricular outflow tract arrhythmias. Circ Arrhythm Electrophysiol 2014;7(4):691–700.

24. Nogami A. Mapping and ablating ventricular premature contractions that trigger ventricular fibrillation: trigger elimination and substrate modification. J Cardiovasc Electrophysiol 2015;26(1):110–5.

25. Boukens BJD, Christoffels VM, Coronel R, et al. Developmental basis for electrophysiological heterogeneity in the ventricular and outflow tract myocardium as a substrate for life-threatening ventricular arrhythmias. Circ Res 2009;104(1):19–31.

26. Lerman BB. Outflow tract ventricular arrhythmias: an update. Trends Cardiovasc Med 2015;25(6):550–8.

27. Kim YR, Nam G-B, Kwon CH, et al. Second coupling interval of nonsustained ventricular tachycardia to distinguish malignant from benign outflow tract ventricular tachycardias. Heart Rhythm 2014;11(12):2222–30.

28. Igarashi M, Tada H, Kurosaki K, et al. Electrocardiographic determinants of the polymorphic QRS morphology in idiopathic right ventricular outflow tract tachycardia. J Cardiovasc Electrophysiol 2012;23(5):521–6.

29. Gerstein WH, Gerstein NS, Sandoval A, et al. Malignant conversion of benign right ventricular outflow track ventricular tachycardia 18 years post-ablation. J Arrhythm 2015;31(4):240–2.

30. Knecht S, Sacher F, Wright M, et al. Long-term follow-up of idiopathic ventricular fibrillation ablation: a multicenter study. J Am Coll Cardiol 2009;54(6):522–8.

31. Takemoto M, Yoshimura H, Ohba Y, et al. Radiofrequency catheter ablation of premature ventricular complexes from right ventricular outflow tract improves left ventricular dilation and clinical status in patients without structural heart disease. J Am Coll Cardiol 2005;45(8):1259–65.

32. Yarlagadda RK, Iwai S, Stein KM, et al. Reversal of cardiomyopathy in patients with repetitive monomorphic ventricular ectopy originating from the right ventricular outflow tract. Circulation 2005;112(8):1092–7.

33. Li D, Fareh S, Leung TK, et al. Promotion of atrial fibrillation by heart failure in dogs: atrial remodeling of a different sort. Circulation 1999;100(1):87–95.

34. Wang Y, Eltit JM, Kaszala K, et al. Cellular mechanism of premature ventricular contraction-induced cardiomyopathy. Heart Rhythm 2014;11(11):2064–72.

35. Qu Z, Xie L-H, Olcese R, et al. Early afterdepolarizations in cardiac myocytes: beyond reduced repolarization reserve. Cardiovasc Res 2013;99(1):6–15.

36. Volders PG, Vos MA, Szabo B, et al. Progress in the understanding of cardiac early afterdepolarizations and torsades de pointes: time to revise current concepts. Cardiovasc Res 2000;46(3):376–92.

37. Ellis ER, Shvilkin A, Josephson ME. Nonreentrant ventricular arrhythmias in patients with structural heart disease unrelated to abnormal myocardial substrate. Heart Rhythm 2014;11(6):946–52.

38. El Kadri M, Yokokawa M, Labounty T, et al. Effect of ablation of frequent premature ventricular complexes on left ventricular function in patients with nonischemic cardiomyopathy. Heart Rhythm 2015;12(4):706–13.

39. Markowitz SM, Weinsaft JW, Waldman L, et al. Reappraisal of cardiac magnetic resonance imaging in idiopathic outflow tract arrhythmias. J Cardiovasc Electrophysiol 2014;25(12):1328–35.

40. Tandri H, Bluemke DA, Ferrari VA, et al. Findings on magnetic resonance imaging of idiopathic right ventricular outflow tachycardia. Am J Cardiol 2004;94(11):1441–5.

Sustained Ventricular Tachycardia in Apparently Normal Hearts
Ablation Should Be the First Step in Management

Joshua D. Moss, MD, Roderick Tung, MD*

KEYWORDS

- Catheter ablation • Ventricular tachycardia • Implantable cardioverter defibrillator
- Antiarrhythmic drugs

KEY POINTS

- Patients without structural heart disease tend to have fewer morphologies of ventricular tachycardia (VT), with automaticity and triggered activity a more common mechanism than re-entry, associated with extremely low risk of sudden death.
- Ablation can be curative in patients with a single morphology of VT that is focal in origin, particularly in patients without overt structural heart disease.
- There are limited data in secondary prevention implantable cardioverter defibrillator (ICD) literature to support the routine implementation of ICD in normal hearts.
- Antiarrhythmic drugs have not been shown to reduce all-cause mortality in patients with or without structural heart disease.
- Data examining the incidence of arrhythmic death in patients with structural heart disease with lower risk features such as tolerated VT and ejection fraction greater than 35% demonstrate a low incidence of annual sudden death. This data may potentially be extrapolated to patients without overt structural heart disease.

Catheter ablation has been demonstrated to be an effective therapy for ventricular arrhythmias across the entire spectrum of patients, with structurally normal hearts to advanced fibrosis with systolic dysfunction.[1,2] In the latter group, ablation is typically performed as an adjunct to antiarrhythmic therapy, with background implantable cardioverter-defibrillator (ICD) therapy. Although ICD is merely an abortive therapy, and antiarrhythmic drug (AAD) therapy is suppressive therapy, catheter ablation is the only curative treatment modality in the armamentarium for ventricular arrhythmias, short of cardiac transplantation. The ideal clinical setting for catheter ablation as a stand-alone therapy is in patient profiles without structural heart disease (SHD) that are at low risk for subsequent sudden death. In this article, the role of catheter ablation as first-line therapy in patients with apparently normal hearts is discussed. The comparative evidence for ICD and effectiveness of

Disclosures/Conflicts of Interest: None.
Center for Arrhythmia Care, Heart and Vascular Center, The University of Chicago Medicine, 5841 South Maryland Avenue, Chicago, IL 60637, USA
* Corresponding author. Center for Arrhythmia Care, The University of Chicago Medicine, 5841 South Maryland Avenue, MC 6080, Chicago, IL 60637.
E-mail address: rodericktung@uchicago.edu

Card Electrophysiol Clin 8 (2016) 623–630
http://dx.doi.org/10.1016/j.ccep.2016.04.011
1877-9182/16/$ – see front matter © 2016 Elsevier Inc. All rights reserved.

antiarrhythmic drugs in patients with normal ejection fraction (EF) are reviewed, as well as highlighted areas of uncertainty-advanced imaging methods have the potential to identify "concealed" or subtle fibrosis and/or inflammation not previously recognized by angiography and echocardiography as "overt" SHD.

COMMON TYPES OF VENTRICULAR TACHYCARDIA IN STRUCTURALLY NORMAL

Sustained ventricular tachycardia (VT) in patients without overt SHD is unrelated to myocardial scar and typically thought to be the result of automaticity or triggered activity. Patients with myocardial scar substrates harbor the ideal scenario for re-entrant mechanisms and typically have multiple circuits, yielding on average 2 to 3 VT morphologies seen during catheter ablation.[3,4] The curative potential for catheter ablation of VT is logically highest in patients with a single focus, represented by a singular electrocardiographic morphology.

In patients without overt SHD, the most common ventricular arrhythmias are the adenosine-sensitive VTs, accounting for approximately 90% of all idiopathic VTs.[5] The mechanism of these arrhythmias is triggered activity due to cyclic adenosine monophosphate mediated-delayed afterdepolarizations, with characteristic features of initiation and termination.[6,7] Two phenotypic forms of adenosine-sensitive VT are commonly described, with the more common presenting as frequent premature ventricular complexes (PVCs), couplets, and salvos of non-sustained VT that often occur at rest or after exercise. The less common form is precipitated by exercise or emotional stress, rather than being suppressed by it, and often presents as sustained VT.

The commonest location of VT in patients without overt SHD, historically called repetitive monomorphic VT, arises from the right ventricular outflow tract (RVOT). In one series, 75% of patients with sustained monomorphic idiopathic VT and 89% of with nonsustained VT were found to have an RVOT site of origin.[8] The arrhythmia classically occurs in younger age with adrenergic triggers, often at peak exercise or during the cool-down period. Sudden death is exceedingly rare, although short-coupled variants resulting in R-on-T phenomenon have been reported with polymorphic VT and ventricular fibrillation in rare cases.[9–11] Ablation success and elimination of this condition can be achieved with a single targeted radiofrequency application. After successful curative ablation, medications are typically discontinued. Structural abnormalities in the right ventricle need to be considered and excluded because the outflow tract comprises 1 of the 3 corners in the "triangle of dysplasia" seen in arrhythmogenic RV cardiomyopathy.[12]

Over the past 10 years, a greater appreciation of outflow tract arrhythmias with precordial lead transition at V3 and earlier on 12-lead ECG has prompted successful mapping and ablation approaches in the aortic root, within the cusps adjacent to the sinuses of Valsalva.[13,14] Focal mechanisms from myocardial fibers at the top of the left ventricular (LV) ostium at the junction of the valves are thought to be the pathophysiologic basis. The risk of sudden death does not appear to be higher compared with patients with RVOT origins. In a recent large-scale, multicenter analysis of outcomes of ablation of idiopathic PVCs, the overall acute success rate was 84%. Success rates were highest (93%) for patients with an RVOT site of origin, with the same patients exhibiting a trend toward the lowest major complication rate (2.1%).[15]

Idiopathic left VT, most commonly arising from the posterior fascicle, is the second most common cause of VT in the absence of overt SHD. Re-entry has been proposed as the common mechanism, with an antegrade limb in a slow verapamil-sensitive zone of the septum with exit and retrograde activation using the fascicle.[16,17] The mechanism of these tachycardias has been demonstrated via entrainment maneuvers.[18–20] This form of VT also has an excellent long-term prognosis,[21,22] although cases of tachycardia-mediated cardiomyopathy and sudden cardiac death have been infrequently reported.[23] VTs originating from the fascicular system are highly curable with ablative therapy, even when the clinical tachycardia cannot be induced and mapped in the electrophysiology laboratory.[24,25] Current guidelines support the primary role for ablation, and ICD implantation is not indicated in this population.

Based on the low overall risk for sudden cardiac death and high success rate of ablative therapy, the 2008 American College of Cardiology/American Heart Association/Heart Rhythm Society Guidelines for Device-based Therapy of Cardiac Rhythm Abnormalities classifies ICD therapy as class III (not indicated) for patients with outflow tract VT, idiopathic VT, or fascicular VT in the absence of SHD.[26] For these abovementioned reasons, catheter ablation is clearly the first-line approach for these VT phenotypes because it is curative in the vast majority of patients.

THE CASE AGAINST IMPLANTABLE CARDIOVERTER-DEFIBRILLATOR AS FIRST-LINE THERAPY

Although an ICD is intuitively useful in preventing arrhythmic death as the most effective abortive therapy for VT, the evidence supporting its role in secondary prevention has important limitations. In the Antiarrhythmics Versus Implantable Defibrillators trial (AVID), patients resuscitated from ventricular fibrillation or VT with syncope, or LV EF 40% or less and symptoms of hemodynamic compromise (syncope, near-syncope, congestive heart failure, angina) caused by the arrhythmia, were randomly assigned to ICD placement or antiarrhythmic drug treatment.[27] The aggregated mortality reduction conferred by the ICD (24.6% vs 35.9% at 3 years) forms a cornerstone of the guidelines for ICD placement for secondary prevention. Although AVID demonstrated a significant reduction in mortality in patients that received an ICD after resuscitated cardiac arrest, the mean prolongation in life was 4 months. Furthermore, there was incomplete and disproportionate β-blocker penetration at the time that this study was performed (38.1% ICD vs 11.0% control at 1 year).

Importantly, in a prespecified subgroup analysis, the benefit from ICD was not observed in patients with EF greater than 35%. The case in favor of secondary prevention ICD implantation is further weakened by the failure of both Canadian Implantable Defibrillator Study and Cardiac Arrest Study Hamburg to demonstrate a significant reduction in mortality in similar populations.[28] In a meta-analysis, patients with EF greater than 35% did not experience survival benefit, which strongly supports the authors' central argument that catheter ablation should be the first-line therapy (**Fig. 1**).

In a retrospective, multivariate analysis of the AVID Registry by Pinski and colleagues,[29] the strongest predictors of mortality in patients who did not receive an ICD included severe left ventricular dysfunction and history of congestive heart failure. The hemodynamic category of the index arrhythmia, whether tolerated or untolerated, did not influence survival. Although a primary conclusion was that tolerated VT in patients with SHD does not have a benign prognosis, it might also be stated that the extent of SHD itself is the primary predictor of both arrhythmias and associated mortality.

A subsequent substudy by Domanski and colleagues[30] further evaluated the influence of baseline EF on the risk of arrhythmic death in this secondary prevention population. In the subset of patients randomized to antiarrhythmic drug treatment who had an EF greater than 40%, the 2-year survival was between 85% and 90%. In multivariate analysis, the risk of arrhythmic death in patients treated with antiarrhythmic drugs rather than an ICD decreased by 39% for every 10% increase in EF (**Fig. 2**). Not surprisingly, the risk of arrhythmic death was relatively low across the entire range of LV function for patients randomized to ICD implant. However, the risk of death from congestive heart failure did decrease significantly with increase in EF, suggesting that the mode of death was indeed adjudicated with reasonable accuracy.

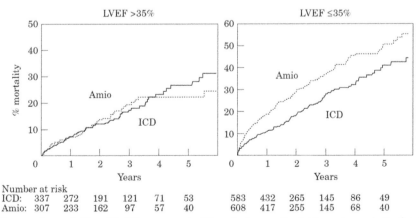

Fig. 1. No difference in mortality with ICD compared with amiodarone (Amio) in meta-analysis of secondary prevention trials in patients with EF greater than 35%. LVEF, left ventricular ejection fraction. (*From* Connolly SJ, Hallstrom AP, Cappato R, et al. Meta-analysis of the implantable cardioverter defibrillator secondary prevention trials. AVID, CASH and CIDS studies. Antiarrhythmics vs implantable defibrillator study. Cardiac Arrest Study Hamburg. Canadian Implantable Defibrillator Study. Eur Heart J 2000;21:2074; with permission.)

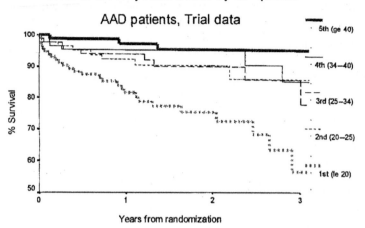

Fig. 2. Gradient in survival based on EF supports the concept that the risk of sudden death is sufficiently low in patients without apparent SHD. AAD, antiarrhythmic drugs.

Despite these weaknesses in the evidence for ICD, a class I indication in the setting of secondary prevention remains in the 2008 ICD guidelines without regard for presence or absence of structural heart disease. In addition, the presence of any spontaneous sustained monomorphic VT with SHD, regardless of EF, is a class I recommendation, which is not fully supported by the analyses of patients with EF greater than 35% in secondary prevention trials. Although ICD therapy is a class IIa recommendation in patients with sustained VT with normal or near-normal ventricular function, the C level of evidence indicates the absence of randomized and non-randomized data. In patients with VTs that are amenable to curative catheter ablation, the relevance of all these recommendations is less clear.

THE CASE AGAINST ANTIARRHYTHMIC MEDICATIONS AS FIRST-LINE THERAPY

As with ICD therapy, it remains intuitive that antiarrhythmic medications should result in a reduction

in mortality. However, trials like the European Myocardial Infarct Amiodarone Trial have suggested a reduction in arrhythmic mortality without an overall favorable impact on all-cause mortality.[31,32] In part, this may be due to the toxicities that are known with amiodarone, which is the most frequently prescribed medication for ventricular arrhythmias. In the Sudden Cardiac Death in Heart Failure Trial (SCD-HeFT), the prescription of amiodarone was harmful when compared with placebo in patients with New York Heart Association (NYHA) class III (1.44, confidence interval 1.05–1.97, P = .01) (Fig. 3).[33] In the Multicenter Unsustained Tachycardia Trial, antiarrhythmic therapy also had a trend toward increased mortality compared with electrophysiology (EP) study-directed ICD therapy.[34]

In the absence of overt SHD, class Ic agents may be preferred to minimize the potential for long-term side effects of amiodarone, although data have shown limited success. The Cardiac

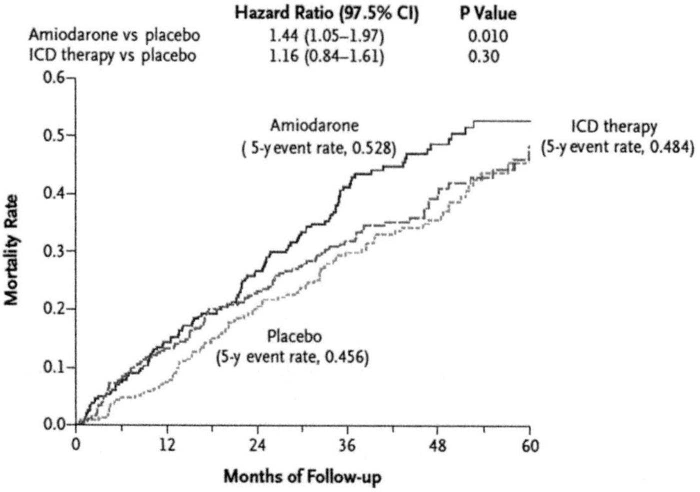

	Hazard Ratio (97.5% CI)	P Value
Amiodarone vs placebo	1.44 (1.05–1.97)	0.010
ICD therapy vs placebo	1.16 (0.84–1.61)	0.30

Fig. 3. Amiodarone was associated with increased mortality relative to placebo in NYHA III patients in SCD-HeFT.

Arrhythmia Suppression Trial highlights the potential role for proarrhythmia in the immediate period after myocardial infarction in patients with ventricular ectopy.[35] To date, there are no data to support the notion that antiarrhythmic medications reduce mortality in patients with VT, in the presence or absence of SHD. Catheter ablation is currently indicated when medications are not desired, effective, or tolerated, but it is the authors' contention that in young patients without SHD, it should not be desired by the physician either if catheter ablation has a high likelihood to be curative.

EXTRAPOLATION OF DATA IN STRUCTURAL HEART DISEASE

The argument for catheter ablation as first-line therapy in patients without overt SHD can be further strengthened by examining studies of ablation without background ICD therapy in higher risk patients with overt and mild SHD. The recently published International Ventricular Tachycardia Center Collaborative Group demonstrated that even in the presence of SHD (EF <50%), elimination of VT with catheter of ablation was strongly associated with improved transplant-free survival in a cohort of 2061 patients.[4] The risk for VT recurrence was nearly 7-fold for transplant and mortality, and it provides support that catheter ablation alone (80% had ICD) may have mortality benefit in patients with overt SHD.

In a multicenter European study by Maury and colleagues,[36] ablation as primary strategy without "backup" ICD was tested among 166 patients with tolerated VT and EF greater than 30% in a mixed population of ischemic cardiomyopathy, nonischemic cardiomyopathy, and arrhythmogenic right ventricular cardiomyopathy. With a control group population of 178 matched during the same period, overall mortality was the same at 12%. Only 2 patients in the ablation group died of arrhythmic causes (2.4%), and most recurrences were nonfatal. The investigators concluded that ablation as first-and-only strategy is clinically feasible and randomized studies are necessary. This provocative data may potentially be extrapolated to a healthier population with normal EF in the presence of mild, subtle, or unapparent disease, where it is biologically plausible that mortalities would be lower.

In a retrospective study published before the ICD era,[37] 124 patients who presented with hemodynamically tolerated VT were followed for a mean of 3 years after either arrhythmia surgery (46 patients) or antiarrhythmic drug treatment (78 patients). Most of these patients had multivessel coronary artery disease and LV systolic dysfunction, and 60% had an LV aneurysm—much less commonly seen in the current era of early revascularization and aggressive medical therapy for LV remodeling. Despite the significant SHD and high overall mortality of 29%, the rate of sudden death was only 2.4% per year on average, and even lower in the surgically treated cohort. Although there are inherent pitfalls in the assignment of a specific cause of death, particularly when being done retrospectively, it is remarkable that the yearly rate of SCD was lower than even the rate of arrhythmic death in the AVID cohort of ICD recipients. Similarly, in unpublished data from the University of Pennsylvania, a cohort of patients who underwent surgical ablation for VT had a high 5-year mortality (nearly 45%), but a low incidence of sudden cardiac death averaging just more than 1% per year.[38]

Thus, even in patients with relatively preserved EF but some SHD, some of whom suffered ventricular fibrillation or poorly tolerated VT, the risk of sudden cardiac death is relatively low. It is reasonable to presume that in the absence of any SHD, and with the current techniques and technologies for ablation of VT and VF brought to bear, the risk would be even lower—perhaps even less than those associated with ICD implant.

PATIENTS WITH INAPPARENT OR "CONCEALED" STRUCTURAL HEART DISEASE

As MRI is increasingly performed at tertiary VT management centers, a greater appreciation of substrates with focal regions of fibrosis in the presence of a preserved EF has emerged. For this reason, the authors believe that MRI is an important, if not essential imaging modality that offers incremental prognostication and risk stratification in patients with normal echocardiography. The case for this assertion may be borrowed from hypertrophic cardiomyopathy literature, where the presence of delayed enhancement may signal higher risk for ventricular arrhythmias and sudden death.[39]

Although the case has been made for ablation as first-line therapy in patients without overt SHD, there is currently no literature with adequate power to provide guidance on those with concealed SHD in the setting of normal EF. Based on observational data that associated larger scar areas with more VT morphologies, it is plausible that smaller scars may be the most amenable to curative ablation. Multiple observational ablation studies in overt SHD demonstrate a gradient in outcomes in relation to extent of scar size.[40–42] However, a study by Wijnmaalen and colleagues[43] examining the role of reperfusion on postmyocardial infarct substrate

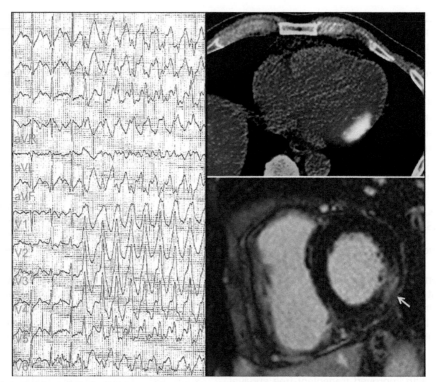

Fig. 4. Evidence of "concealed" SHD in an otherwise healthy patient with normal EF presenting with nonoutflow VT morphology seen on exercise treadmill. Yellow arrow indicates delayed enhancement.

characteristics found an association between smaller scars and faster VTs.

In addition to fibrosis, inflammation may play an important role in ventricular arrhythmogenesis. A recent report by Kandolin and colleagues[44] demonstrated a 20 times increase in incidence of sarcoidosis over a 25- year period, which is likely due to improvements in clinical awareness, suspicion, and refinements in imaging technology. In a 3-year series of 103 patients presenting for VT management at University of California, Los Angeles, the authors reported that nearly 50% demonstrated focal abnormalities on fasting fludeoxyglucose F 18 scans, suggesting that a large proportion of patients have arrhythmogenic inflammatory cardiomyopathy.[45] The treatment of these patients involves an additional layer of complexity, as immunosuppressive therapy and disease-specific medical therapies in the cases of biopsy-proved sarcoidosis should be first-line therapy. **Fig. 4** shows a patient with concealed SHD with apparently normal ejection fraction and sustained VT, with abnormalities on PET and MRI consistent with the suspected origin of sustained monomorphic VT seen on treadmill testing.

Future directions in the field require observational and prospective data on this emerging population of concealed SHD. As ICD would not typically be recommended in a primary prevention setting, these scenarios may be an optimal arena to test the effectiveness of primary ablation therapy. However, a relatively low incidence of this phenotype in patients who present with VT may limit the power to plan future studies. This limitation may be counterbalanced by increased recognition of concealed disease, due to increase awareness and resolution of advanced imaging modalities.

SUMMARY

In summary, there is a paucity of data to support the notion that either ICD therapy or antiarrhythmic therapy has a favorable impact on all-cause mortality in patients with VT and EF greater than 35%, and both therapies are associated with real risks. Extrapolation of the literature in healthier subgroups of patients with SHD to a population without apparent SHD seems reasonable and translates to a sufficiently low rate of sudden death and overall mortality. ICD therapy is a class III recommendation in patients with idiopathic VT, outflow tract VT, and fascicular VT because ablation is typically curative in these phenotypes. Catheter ablation is optimally positioned to be the first and preferred therapy for patients that have no apparent or overt SHD because the risk of sudden death is low, even in the event of procedural failure. Further studies are necessary to evaluate the risk of sudden death in patients with concealed SHD revealed only on MRI and PET.

REFERENCES

1. Aliot EM, Stevenson WG, Almendral-Garrote JM, et al. EHRA/HRS expert consensus on catheter ablation of ventricular arrhythmias: developed in a partnership with the European Heart Rhythm Association (EHRA), a registered branch of the European Society of Cardiology (ESC), and the Heart Rhythm Society (HRS); in collaboration with the American College of Cardiology (ACC) and the American Heart Association (AHA). Heart Rhythm 2009;6:886–933.

2. Pedersen CT, Kay GN, Kalman J, et al. EHRA/HRS/APHRS expert consensus on ventricular arrhythmias. Heart Rhythm 2014;11:e166–96.

3. Stevenson WG, Friedman PL, Kocovic D, et al. Radiofrequency catheter ablation of ventricular tachycardia after myocardial infarction. Circulation 1998;98:308–14.

4. Tung R, Vaseghi M, Frankel DS, et al. Freedom from recurrent ventricular tachycardia after catheter ablation is associated with improved survival in patients with structural heart disease: an International VT Ablation Center Collaborative Group study. Heart Rhythm 2015;12:1997–2007.

5. Issa ZF, Miller JM, Zipes DP. Clinical arrhythmology and electrophysiology: a companion to Braunwald's heart disease. Philadelphia: Saunders; 2009.

6. Iwai S, Cantillon DJ, Kim RJ, et al. Right and left ventricular outflow tract tachycardias: evidence for a common electrophysiologic mechanism. J Cardiovasc Electrophysiol 2006;17:1052–8.

7. Lerman BB, Stein KM, Markowitz SM. Mechanisms of idiopathic left ventricular tachycardia. J Cardiovasc Electrophysiol 1997;8:571–83.

8. Kim RJ, Iwai S, Markowitz SM, et al. Clinical and electrophysiological spectrum of idiopathic ventricular outflow tract arrhythmias. J Am Coll Cardiol 2007; 49:2035–43.

9. Noda T, Shimizu W, Taguchi A, et al. Malignant entity of idiopathic ventricular fibrillation and polymorphic ventricular tachycardia initiated by premature extrasystoles originating from the right ventricular outflow tract. J Am Coll Cardiol 2005;46:1288–94.

10. Viskin S, Rosso R, Rogowski O, et al. The "short-coupled" variant of right ventricular outflow ventricular tachycardia: a not-so-benign form of benign ventricular tachycardia? J Cardiovasc Electrophysiol 2005;16:912–6.

11. Bottoni N, Quartieri F, Lolli G, et al. Sudden death in a patient with idiopathic right ventricular outflow tract arrhythmia. J Cardiovasc Med (Hagerstown) 2009; 10:801–3.

12. Corrado D, Wichter T, Link MS, et al. Treatment of arrhythmogenic right ventricular cardiomyopathy/dysplasia: an international task force consensus statement. Circulation 2015;132:441–53.

13. Ouyang F, Fotuhi P, Ho SY, et al. Repetitive monomorphic ventricular tachycardia originating from the aortic sinus cusp: electrocardiographic characterization for guiding catheter ablation. J Am Coll Cardiol 2002;39:500–8.

14. Yamada T, Yoshida N, Murakami Y, et al. Electrocardiographic characteristics of ventricular arrhythmias originating from the junction of the left and right coronary sinuses of Valsalva in the aorta: the activation pattern as a rationale for the electrocardiographic characteristics. Heart Rhythm 2008;5:184–92.

15. Latchamsetty R, Yokokawa M, Morady F, et al. Multicenter outcomes for catheter ablation of idiopathic premature ventricular complexes. J Am Coll Cardiol: Clinical Electophysiology 2015;1:116–23.

16. Nogami A, Naito S, Tada H, et al. Verapamil-sensitive left anterior fascicular ventricular tachycardia: results of radiofrequency ablation in six patients. J Cardiovasc Electrophysiol 1998;9:1269–78.

17. Nogami A, Naito S, Tada H, et al. Demonstration of diastolic and presystolic Purkinje potentials as critical potentials in a macroreentry circuit of verapamil-sensitive idiopathic left ventricular tachycardia. J Am Coll Cardiol 2000;36:811–23.

18. Zipes DP, Foster PR, Troup PJ, et al. Atrial induction of ventricular tachycardia: reentry versus triggered automaticity. Am J Cardiol 1979;44:1–8.

19. Lin FC, Finley CD, Rahimtoola SH, et al. Idiopathic paroxysmal ventricular tachycardia with a QRS pattern of right bundle branch block and left axis deviation: a unique clinical entity with specific properties. Am J Cardiol 1983;52:95–100.

20. Maruyama M, Tadera T, Miyamoto S, et al. Demonstration of the reentrant circuit of verapamil-sensitive idiopathic left ventricular tachycardia: direct evidence for macroreentry as the underlying mechanism. J Cardiovasc Electrophysiol 2001;12: 968–72.

21. Lemery R, Brugada P, Bella PD, et al. Nonischemic ventricular tachycardia. Clinical course and long-term follow-up in patients without clinically overt heart disease. Circulation 1989;79:990–9.

22. Ohe T, Aihara N, Kamakura S, et al. Long-term outcome of verapamil-sensitive sustained left ventricular tachycardia in patients without structural heart disease. J Am Coll Cardiol 1995;25:54–8.

23. Toivonen L, Nieminen M. Persistent ventricular tachycardia resulting in left ventricular dilatation treated with verapamil. Int J Cardiol 1986;13:361–5.

24. Nakagawa H, Beckman KJ, McClelland JH, et al. Radiofrequency catheter ablation of idiopathic left ventricular tachycardia guided by a Purkinje potential. Circulation 1993;88:2607–17.

25. Lin D, Hsia HH, Gerstenfeld EP, et al. Idiopathic fascicular left ventricular tachycardia: linear ablation lesion strategy for noninducible or nonsustained tachycardia. Heart Rhythm 2005;2:934–9.

26. Epstein AE, Dimarco JP, Ellenbogen KA, et al. ACC/AHA/HRS 2008 guidelines for device-based therapy of cardiac rhythm abnormalities. Heart Rhythm 2008;5:e1–62.

27. A comparison of antiarrhythmic-drug therapy with implantable defibrillators in patients resuscitated from near-fatal ventricular arrhythmias. The antiarrhythmics versus implantable defibrillators (AVID) investigators. N Engl J Med 1997;337:1576–83.

28. Connolly SJ, Hallstrom AP, Cappato R, et al. Meta-analysis of the implantable cardioverter defibrillator secondary prevention trials. AVID, CASH and CIDS studies. Antiarrhythmics Vs Implantable Defibrillator study. Cardiac Arrest Study Hamburg. Canadian Implantable Defibrillator Study. Eur Heart J 2000; 21:2071–8.

29. Pinski SL, Yao Q, Epstein AE, et al. Determinants of outcome in patients with sustained ventricular tachyarrhythmias: the antiarrhythmics versus implantable defibrillators (AVID) study registry. Am Heart J 2000;139:804–13.

30. Domanski MJ, Epstein A, Hallstrom A, et al. Survival of antiarrhythmic or implantable cardioverter defibrillator treated patients with varying degrees of left ventricular dysfunction who survived malignant ventricular arrhythmias. J Cardiovasc Electrophysiol 2002;13:580–3.

31. Julian DG, Camm AJ, Frangin G, et al. Randomised trial of effect of amiodarone on mortality in patients with left-ventricular dysfunction after recent myocardial infarction: EMIAT. European Myocardial Infarct Amiodarone Trial Investigators. Lancet 1997;349: 667–74.

32. Julian DG. The amiodarone trials. Eur Heart J 1997; 18:1361–2.

33. Bardy GH, Lee KL, Mark DB, et al. Amiodarone or an implantable cardioverter-defibrillator for congestive heart failure. N Engl J Med 2005;352:225–37.

34. Buxton AE, Lee KL, Fisher JD, et al. A randomized study of the prevention of sudden death in patients with coronary artery disease. Multicenter Unsustained Tachycardia Trial Investigators. N Engl J Med 1999;341:1882–90.

35. Preliminary report: effect of encainide and flecainide on mortality in a randomized trial of arrhythmia suppression after myocardial infarction. The Cardiac Arrhythmia Suppression Trial (CAST) investigators. N Engl J Med 1989;321:406–12.

36. Maury P, Baratto F, Zeppenfeld K, et al. Radio-frequency ablation as primary management of well-tolerated sustained monomorphic ventricular tachycardia in patients with structural heart disease and left ventricular ejection fraction over 30%. Eur Heart J 2014;35:1479–85.

37. Sarter BH, Finkle JK, Gerszten RE, et al. What is the risk of sudden cardiac death in patients presenting with hemodynamically stable sustained ventricular tachycardia after myocardial infarction? J Am Coll Cardiol 1996;28:122–9.

38. Almendral J, Josephson ME. All patients with hemodynamically tolerated postinfarction ventricular tachycardia do not require an implantable cardioverter-defibrillator. Circulation 2007;116:1204–12.

39. Rubinshtein R, Glockner JF, Ommen SR, et al. Characteristics and clinical significance of late gadolinium enhancement by contrast-enhanced magnetic resonance imaging in patients with hypertrophic cardiomyopathy. Circ Heart Fail 2010;3:51–8.

40. Arenal A, Hernandez J, Calvo D, et al. Safety, long-term results, and predictors of recurrence after complete endocardial ventricular tachycardia substrate ablation in patients with previous myocardial infarction. Am J Cardiol 2013;111:499–505.

41. Dinov B, Schratter A, Schirripa V, et al. Procedural outcomes and survival after catheter ablation of ventricular tachycardia in relation to electroanatomical substrate in patients with nonischemic-dilated cardiomyopathy: the role of unipolar voltage mapping. J Cardiovasc Electrophysiol 2015. [Epub ahead of print].

42. Di Marco A, Paglino G, Oloriz T, et al. Impact of a chronic total occlusion in an infarct-related artery on the long-term outcome of ventricular tachycardia ablation. J Cardiovasc Electrophysiol 2015; 26:532–9.

43. Wijnmaalen AP, Schalij MJ, von der Thusen JH, et al. Early reperfusion during acute myocardial infarction affects ventricular tachycardia characteristics and the chronic electroanatomic and histological substrate. Circulation 2010;121:1887–95.

44. Kandolin R, Lehtonen J, Airaksinen J, et al. Cardiac sarcoidosis: epidemiology, characteristics, and outcome over 25 years in a nationwide study. Circulation 2015;131:624–32.

45. Tung R, Bauer B, Schelbert H, et al. Incidence of abnormal positron emission tomography in patients with unexplained cardiomyopathy and ventricular arrhythmias: the potential role of occult inflammation in arrhythmogenesis. Heart Rhythm 2015;12:2488–98.

Sustained Ventricular Tachycardia in Apparently Normal Hearts

Medical Therapy Should be the First Step in Management

Ali Kazemi Saeid, MD, George J. Klein, MD, FHRS, Peter Leong-Sit, MD, MSc, FHRS*

KEYWORDS

• Ventricular tachycardia • Premature ventricular complexes • Medical therapy • Catheter ablation

KEY POINTS

- Idiopathic VT has a favorable prognosis and treatments based on symptom burden should be offered with appropriate care.
- Medical therapies for some forms of idiopathic VT may be less effective than catheter ablation, but carry a reasonable efficacy and suitable safety record appropriate for first-line therapy.
- Although catheter ablation is an effective and reasonably safe therapy, it does carry some risk and should be considered carefully when treating relatively benign conditions, such as idiopathic VT.

INTRODUCTION

Ventricular tachycardia (VT) occurring in structurally normal hearts, without significant ventricular dysfunction or myocardial scar, is referred to as idiopathic VT. The prevalence of idiopathic VT is estimated at 7% to 38% of all patients referred for evaluation of VT.[1]

The causes of idiopathic VT are classified in the following manner: outflow tract VT, fascicular VT, intramural VT, annular VT, and epicardial VT. Fig. 1 shows an anatomic-based classification of the various forms of idiopathic VT. By far, the most common etiologies of idiopathic VT are outflow tract and fascicular VT. These account for approximately 90% of all idiopathic VT.

Although the mechanisms of the various forms of idiopathic VT are different and include cAMP-mediated delayed afterdepolarizations, automaticity, and microreentry for outflow tract VT[2] and macroreentry for some forms of fascicular VT,[3] one common defining feature of all causes of idiopathic VT is that they share a favorable prognosis. Because of the high prevalence and increased mortality risk of VT in the context of structural heart disease, there have been extensive clinical trials and cohort studies on the treatment and management of VT associated with cardiomyopathy. The same cannot be said for idiopathic VT, which is less prevalent and is associated with a favorable prognosis. Therefore, guidelines for treatment are based on the known complications associated with idiopathic VT, the efficacy and risks of medical therapies, and the relative efficacy and risks of invasive therapies.

CURRENT GUIDELINES

As a starting point, the most recent American College of Cardiology/American Heart Association/European Society of Cardiology guidelines

Western University, London, Ontario, Canada
* Corresponding author. Division of Cardiology, Department of Medicine, 339 Windermere Road, Office C6-113, London, Ontario N6A 5A5, Canada.
E-mail address: pleongs@uwo.ca

Card Electrophysiol Clin 8 (2016) 631–639
http://dx.doi.org/10.1016/j.ccep.2016.04.012
1877-9182/16/$ – see front matter © 2016 Elsevier Inc. All rights reserved.

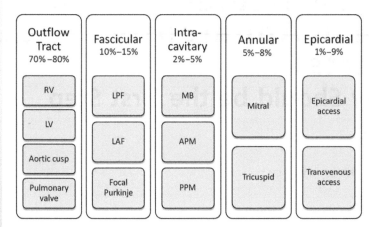

Fig. 1. Classification and prevalence of idiopathic VT. APM, anterior papillary muscle; LAF, left anterior fascicle; LPF, left posterior fascicule; LV, left ventricle; MB, moderator band; PPM, posterior papillary muscle; RV, right ventricle.

for the management of ventricular arrhythmias date back to 2006[4] with an expert consensus update by the European Heart Rhythm Association/Heart Rhythm Society/Asia Pacific Heart Rhythm Society in 2014[5] and a European Society of Cardiology guideline from 2015.[6] The European Heart Rhythm Association/Heart Rhythm Society/Asia Pacific Heart Rhythm Society expert consensus update suggests that the primary indication for treatment of sustained idiopathic VT is largely based on symptoms. It offers three main options, which are all reasonable: (1) pharmacologic therapy with β-blockade or nondihydropyridine calcium channel blockade; (2) antiarrhythmic therapy with sotalol, flecainide, mexiletine, propafenone, or amiodarone; or (3) catheter ablation. They do not recommend a specific first-line therapy but highlight that low-risk drugs, such as β-blockade and calcium channel blockade, have modest efficacy; that more effective antiarrhythmic medications carry a greater side effect profile; and that the efficacy of catheter ablation largely depends on the inducibility of the arrhythmia.

However, the European Society of Cardiology 2015 guidelines favor a slightly less invasive approach citing a Class I recommendation with Level B evidence that catheter ablation for right ventricle outflow tract VT should only be performed in symptomatic patients failing antiarrhythmic drug therapy or with a decline in left ventricle (LV) function. Moreover, for higher risk etiologies of idiopathic VT (eg, LV outflow tract, aortic cusp VT, or epicardial VT), sodium channel blockers are recommended as the therapy of choice with catheter ablation only as an option for experienced operators after drug therapy has failed. We now explore the evidence and rationale behind these recommendations.

IDIOPATHIC VENTRICULAR TACHYCARDIA HAS A FAVORABLE PROGNOSIS

In determining the best course of action for a patient with any diagnosis, the potential treatments must be weighed carefully by comparing their relative risks with their potential for efficacy. Perhaps more importantly, these risks and benefits must first be weighed against the potential for harm of the diagnosis itself. For instance, when dealing with high-risk diagnoses, such as lung cancer, one accepts toxic and high-risk treatments, such as chemotherapy and radiation therapy. Idiopathic VT, fortunately, does not portend the same level of mortality or morbidity.

The most common form of idiopathic VT, outflow tract VT, is known to have a benign natural history. Long-term data on 133 patients with sustained outflow tract VT and a median follow-up of 11.3 years (range, 29–248 years) demonstrated that with no invasive treatments, there were zero deaths from cardiac disease.[7] Similarly, with the second most common form of idiopathic VT, fascicular VT, the long-term prognosis is equally favorable with zero cardiac deaths among 33 patients followed for a mean of 5.7 ± 4.7 years in one cohort[8] and only one unexplained death in another cohort of 37 patients followed for 5.8 years (range, 1–13 years).[9] The less common etiologies of idiopathic VT, such as papillary muscle, moderator band, annular, and epicardial, have no reported long-term data, but have not been reported to be associated with malignant outcomes.

Although there are reports of uncommon malignant forms of idiopathic VT, such as short-coupled outflow tract premature ventricular complexes leading to polymorphic VT,[10] there are clinical features that identify these exceptional patients who require more attention and more aggressive management. Such features include a short coupling interval of initiating premature ventricular complexes, a slightly wider QRS, a shorter tachycardia cycle length, and the presence of polymorphic VT.[11,12]

Hence, for most patients with idiopathic VT, treatment is based on symptom burden and quality of life. In this context, it is prudent that they are offered the simplest and safest strategies first, rather than the most effective. After all, failed safe first-line therapies can always be escalated to second-line therapies.

MEDICAL THERAPIES FOR IDIOPATHIC VENTRICULAR TACHYCARDIA ARE REASONABLY EFFECTIVE

For outflow tract VT, medical therapies have been well established. Lerman and colleagues[13] have shown that most forms of outflow tract VT are sensitive to adenosine and the most likely mechanism is catecholamine-mediated delayed afterdepolarizations and triggered activity. For chronic management, β-blockade has been demonstrated to have reasonable efficacy likely because of the role of sympathovagal balance in the initiation of outflow tract VT.[14] In a randomized, placebo-controlled trial, it was shown that atenolol improved symptoms and reduced the ventricular ectopy count in patients with symptomatic ventricular arrhythmia without structural heart disease.[15]

Therapy with sodium-channel blockers and potassium-channel blockers seems to be more effective than β-blockers for outflow tract VT.[16] In longer term follow-up, treatment with agents, such as flecainide, propafenone, sotalol, or metoprolol, led to successful symptomatic suppression in 48% of the patients.[7] Most of these patients (73%) had spontaneous resolution and were able to discontinue the agents within 20 months while remaining symptom-free. The unusually high spontaneous resolution rate seen in this particular study speaks to the importance of patient selection when deciding who may need medical or invasive treatments. At the same time, the high spontaneous resolution rate may indicate that this study may overestimate the true efficacy of antiarrhythmic medications.

The sensitivity of fascicular VT to calcium channel blockade is also well established with an excellent response rate in small case series.[17,18] In the largest case series of 37 patients, verapamil repeatedly terminated episodes of VT in 100% of patients. Among the 37 patients, 14 (37.8%) eventually did not require any chronic medical therapy for the VT, 23 (54.1%) were successfully treated with verapamil, and six (16.2%) had an inadequate response requiring invasive therapies.[9]

Medical treatment of the other causes of idiopathic VT, such as annular and epicardial VT, is not well established, but empiric treatments with β-blockers, sodium channel blockers, and potassium channel blockers have been described.[6]

MEDICAL THERAPIES ARE SAFE

The safety of calcium channel blockade and β-blockade is clear given their ubiquitous use for a variety of chronic conditions, such as hypertension, coronary disease, and cardiomyopathy. Certainly, there are potential side effects when using such medications, such as lightheadedness, fatigue, hypotension, and bradycardia. However, most tolerate these commonly used therapies.

When escalating the medical therapy to sodium channel blockers or potassium channel blockers, there is an elevation in the risk profile of these medications that coincides with the increased efficacy. Although generally safe in a population lacking structural heart disease, such antiarrhythmics are also associated with a small proarrhythmic risk. Safety data from a randomized trial of 200 patients on flecainide or propafenone in a population with atrial fibrillation and no structural heart disease demonstrated three proarrhythmic events with one patient (0.5%) having VT and two patients (1.0%) having atrial fibrillation with rapid rates.[19]

Because of the clear safety profile of β-blockers and calcium channel blockers, and the reasonable safety profile of antiarrhythmic agents in the context of structurally normal hearts, it is challenging to argue against a first-line trial of medical therapies when treating a prognostically benign condition. Recall that approximately half of patients with outflow tract VT and approximately 85% of patients with fascicular VT were treated successfully with medications. Also recall that approximately 75% of the 48% of patients with no recurrences on medications for outflow tract VT and approximately 35% of patients on medications for fascicular VT eventually stopped their medications with spontaneous resolution of their symptoms and no recurrence. If an aggressive first-line cardiac ablation strategy was used, all these patients would have undergone an unnecessary invasive procedure.

CATHETER ABLATION FOR MANY FORMS OF IDIOPATHIC VENTRICULAR TACHYCARDIA IS INEFFECTIVE

Catheter ablation for all forms of idiopathic VT has been demonstrated and reported in terms of proof of concept. The success and recurrence rates largely depend on the experience of the operator, the accessibility of the tachycardia origin, the ease of inducibility of the VT, and the definition of end points. The true efficacy of catheter ablation for idiopathic VT is difficult to determine because the literature is based primarily on cohort studies. Of course, cohort studies may either falsely underestimate the true efficacy of catheter ablation (ie, because of selection bias only the most severe cases undergo ablation) or, conversely, may falsely overestimate the true efficacy (ie, many of the patients may have otherwise had a spontaneous resolution of their symptoms as other cohort studies have suggested).

Despite these limitations, catheter ablation seems to be effective for various forms of idiopathic VT (**Table 1**). For sustained outflow tract VT, the earliest reports of long-term follow-up were from Morady and colleagues.[20] They reported a recurrence after catheter ablation in 2 of 10 patients after a mean follow-up of 33 ± 18 months. A review of success rates using more contemporary ablation techniques found that among 815 patients who underwent ablation of outflow tract VT, the acute efficacy varied from 76% to 100% with a recurrence rate of 0% to 23% after a mean follow-up of between 13 ± 10 months and 56 ± 31 months across eight studies.[21] Furthermore, in a randomized controlled trial comparing catheter ablation with either metoprolol or propafenone for outflow tract ventricular ectopy, catheter ablation was clearly superior with respect to efficacy.[22] In a multicenter study of 1185 patients with ablation for idiopathic ventricular ectopy, a right ventricle outflow tract location was a clear predictor of procedural success (odds ratio, 3.78; 95% confidence interval, 1.87–7.6; $P<.01$).[23]

For fascicular VT, only 42 patients were reported across four studies.[24–27] Catheter ablation was successful acutely in 85% to 100% and the recurrence rate ranged from 0% to 25% after a mean follow-up of between 7 ± 8 months and 16 ± 8 months.[21] For the two most common forms of idiopathic VT, outflow tract and fascicular, the ablation success rates are favorable.

However, the same review of contemporary ablation summarized the efficacy in the less common forms of idiopathic VT.[21] There was a clear theme of high acute success, but a high recurrence rate. Catheter ablation for intracavitary VT was reported in 96 patients across four studies.[28–31] The acute success rate was found to be 89% to 100%, but the recurrence rate was high at 42% to 100% for posterior papillary muscle VT after a follow-up of 0 ± 5 months and 21 ± 9 months. Moderator band VT also had a high recurrence rate of 40% after a follow-up of

22 ± 12 months. Catheter ablation for perivalvular VT in 81 patients across three studies showed acute success rates of 66% to 100%, but a recurrence rate of 81% to 100% after a follow-up period of between 21 ± 15 months and 31 ± 7 months.[32–34] Catheter ablation for epicardial VT in 69 patients across three studies demonstrated acute success in 44% to 100% with recurrence rates of 75% to 100% over a follow-up period of 6 ± 4 months and 31 ± 21 months.[35–37] An epicardial source has been shown to be a clear negative predictor of procedural success (odds ratio, 0.49; 95% confidence interval, 0.27–0.91; $P = .02$).[23]

It is clear from the nonrandomized data that there is a high recurrence rate of VT for intramural, annular, and epicardial VT. Although the high recurrence rates may partly be explained by selection bias (most of these studies included patients who have already failed several antiarrhythmic medications), and although there is reasonable proof of concept that catheter ablation is an option for such patients, it raises large concern to attempt an invasive procedure as a first-line therapy when recurrence rates may be 100% in select populations for some mechanisms of idiopathic VT.

THERE ARE REAL RISKS WITH CATHETER ABLATION

However, arguments could be made for first-line therapy for ablation of outflow tract and fascicular VT given the high rate of efficacy if risks are negligible or at least on par with those associated with the use of β-blockers, calcium channel blockers, or antiarrhythmic medications. Unfortunately, that does not seem to be the case. Katz and colleagues[38] reported on the safety and adverse events of 9699 hospitalizations with VT ablation. In this diverse population, adverse events were reported in 825 patients (8.5%) and included death, stroke, intracerebral hemorrhage, pericardial complications, hematoma or hemorrhage, blood transfusion, or cardiogenic shock. Major adverse events defined as stroke, tamponade, or death occurred in 295 patients (3.0%) with death in 110 (1.1%).

More relevant to a discussion surrounding idiopathic VT, the cohort of patients in this study without structural heart disease included 6635 (68%) of the total hospitalizations. Expectedly, the complication rates were modestly better, but not negligible. Adverse events occurred in 5.6% of hospitalizations, major adverse events in 1.4%, and death occurred in 0.3%. In another multicenter study of 1185 patients undergoing ablation for idiopathic ventricular arrhythmia, the

Table 1
Efficacy of ablation in various forms of idiopathic VT

	Number of Studies (Range of Publication, y)	Total Number of Patients (Range of Patients in Individual Studies)	Range of Mean Age (y)	Range of Follow-Up (mo)	Range of Acute Success (%)	Range of Recurrence at End of Follow-Up (%)
Outflow tract VT[43-50]	8 (2002–2010)	815 (33–168)	39 ± 9, 56 ± 15	13 ± 10, 72 ± 28	76–100	0–23
Fascicular VT[24-27]	4 (1993–2005)	42 (6–120)	24 ± 7, 28 ± 8	7 ± 8, 16 ± 8	85–100	0–25
Intracavitary VT[28-31]	4 (2008–2015)	96 (7–71)	42 ± 13, 47 ± 23	8 ± 4, 22 ± 12	89–100	0–71
Perivalvular VT[32-34]	3 (2005–2011)	81 (19–38)	44 ± 16, 61 ± 14	21 ± 15, 31 ± 7	66–100	0–19
Epicardial VT[35-37]	3 (2009–2015)	69 (4–47)	53 ± 12, 57 ± 19	6 ± 4, 31 ± 21	44–100	0–25

Adapted from Tanawuttiwat T, Nazarian S, Calkins H. The role of catheter ablation in the management of ventricular tachycardia. Eur Heart J 2016;37(7):597.

major complication rate was 2.4% with primarily vascular complications (1.3%) and tamponade (0.8%). **Table 2** demonstrates the complication rates from a single center cohort study and the multicenter study.[23,39]

According to an administrative database of hospitalizations for VT ablation, complications associated with VT ablation seemed to be increasing, rather than decreasing, during recent years.[38] As highlighted in the discussion by Katz and colleagues,[38] the reason for this trend may potentially be explained by an increase in case complexity as VT ablation volumes have increased. There was also an association with higher adverse events in low-volume centers. Should management of idiopathic VT with cardiac ablation become a first-line therapy, the likely unintended consequence would be an increase in the number of low-volume centers performing the procedures. Hence, the reported adverse event rates in the current high-volume expert centers may underestimate the true risks with such a strategy.

CHOOSING MEDICAL THERAPIES AS A FIRST-LINE STRATEGY FOR IDIOPATHIC VENTRICULAR TACHYCARDIA DOES NOT MEAN ELIMINATING THE ROLE OF CATHETER ABLATION

It deserves emphasis that many of the patients included in the cohort studies demonstrating efficacy for catheter ablation have previously failed medical therapies. The common strategy of first attempting a low-cost and safe therapy first, and then escalating therapies to invasive ones for those who fail to respond or who have side effects from the medications seems absolutely sensible. In this context, it is not relevant whether catheter ablation has a superior efficacy compared with medications. Rather, any patient who has success with medications could avoid the cost and risks of an invasive procedure. The threshold for proceeding to invasive therapies can be very low, depending on operator experience and comfort, and depending on patient safety characteristics, preferences, and symptom severity.

APPARENT EXCEPTIONS TO THE RULE

In patients with a high burden of VT or ventricular ectopy, there is a well-described risk of tachycardia-induced cardiomyopathy.[40,41] In this population, catheter ablation has been shown in a nonrandomized cohort to have efficacy in reducing the ectopy burden and improving (although not normalizing) the left ventricular ejection fraction.[42] Moreover, in the context of reduced LV function, the use of many antiarrhythmic agents becomes higher risk. For these reasons, a patient with idiopathic VT who has developed a cardiomyopathy should be treated aggressively and likely with first-line catheter ablation. It should be noted that a patient with tachycardia cardiomyopathy no longer has "an apparently normal heart" and, therefore, is not the focus of this review.

SUMMARY

Idiopathic VT has a favorable prognosis and, therefore, treatments based on symptom burden should be offered with appropriate care. Medical therapies, although perhaps less effective than catheter ablation in some forms of idiopathic VT, carry a reasonable efficacy and a suitable safety record appropriate for a first-line therapy for a relatively benign condition. For some less common forms of idiopathic VT, such as papillary muscle, moderator band, annular, and epicardial VT, recurrence rates may be 100%. In large administrative databases, the risks of catheter ablation are not inconsequential and may only increase with more ubiquitous use in less experienced centers. These findings lead to the conclusion that in patients with VT and a structurally normal heart, medical treatments are absolutely the correct first choice based on safety, effectiveness, and reasonable cost.

Table 2
Prevalence of major complications after radiofrequency ablation

Major Complications	Occurrence, %
Vascular injury	1.3–1.6
Pseudoaneurysm	0.7
Hematoma	0.34
Arteriovenous fistula	0.25
Cardiac tamponade	0.8
Thromboembolism	0.4
Conduction system damage	0.1–0.4
Injury to the coronary arteries	Rare

Adapted from Latchamsetty R, Yokokawa M, Morady F, et al. Multicenter outcomes for catheter ablation of idiopathic premature ventricular complexes. J Am Coll Cardiol: Clin Electrophysiol 2015;1(3):121, with permission; and Peichl P, Wichterle D, Pavlu L, et al. Complications of catheter ablation of ventricular tachycardia: a single-center experience. Circ Arrhythm Electrophysiol 2014;7(4):686.

REFERENCES

1. Hoffmayer KS, Gerstenfeld EP. Diagnosis and management of idiopathic ventricular tachycardia. Curr Probl Cardiol 2013;38(4):131–58.

2. Schlotthauer K, Bers DM. Sarcoplasmic reticulum Ca(2+) release causes myocyte depolarization. Underlying mechanism and threshold for triggered action potentials. Circ Res 2000;87(9):774–80.

3. Ohe T, Shimomura K, Aihara N, et al. Idiopathic sustained left ventricular tachycardia: clinical and electrophysiologic characteristics. Circulation 1988; 77(3):560–8.

4. Zipes DP, Camm AJ, Borggrefe M, et al. ACC/AHA/ESC 2006 guidelines for management of patients with ventricular arrhythmias and the prevention of sudden cardiac death: a report of the American College of Cardiology/American Heart Association task force and the European Society of Cardiology Committee for practice guidelines (writing committee to develop guidelines for management of patients with ventricular arrhythmias and the prevention of sudden cardiac death): developed in collaboration with the European Heart Rhythm Association and the Heart Rhythm Society. Circulation 2006;114(10): e385–484.

5. Pedersen CT, Kay GN, Kalman J, et al. EHRA/HRS/ APHRS expert consensus on ventricular arrhythmias. Heart Rhythm 2014;11(10):e166–96.

6. Priori SG, Blomstrom-Lundqvist C, Mazzanti A, et al. 2015 ESC guidelines for the management of patients with ventricular arrhythmias and the prevention of sudden cardiac death: the task force for the management of patients with ventricular arrhythmias and the prevention of sudden cardiac death of the European Society of Cardiology (ESC)Endorsed by: Association for European Paediatric and Congenital Cardiology (AEPC). Eur Heart J 2015; 36(41):2793–867.

7. Ventura R, Steven D, Klemm HU, et al. Decennial follow-up in patients with recurrent tachycardia originating from the right ventricular outflow tract: electrophysiologic characteristics and response to treatment. Eur Heart J 2007;28(19):2338–45.

8. Gaita F, Giustetto C, Leclercq JF, et al. Idiopathic verapamil-responsive left ventricular tachycardia: clinical characteristics and long-term follow-up of 33 patients. Eur Heart J 1994;15(9):1252–60.

9. Ohe T, Aihara N, Kamakura S, et al. Long-term outcome of verapamil-sensitive sustained left ventricular tachycardia in patients without structural heart disease. J Am Coll Cardiol 1995; 25(1):54–8.

10. Viskin S, Rosso R, Rogowski O, et al. The "short-coupled" variant of right ventricular outflow ventricular tachycardia: a not-so-benign form of benign ventricular tachycardia? J Cardiovasc Electrophysiol 2005;16(8):912–6.

11. Noda T, Shimizu W, Taguchi A, et al. Malignant entity of idiopathic ventricular fibrillation and polymorphic ventricular tachycardia initiated by premature extrasystoles originating from the right ventricular outflow tract. J Am Coll Cardiol 2005; 46(7):1288–94.

12. Shimizu W. Arrhythmias originating from the right ventricular outflow tract: how to distinguish "malignant" from "benign"? Heart Rhythm 2009;6(10): 1507–11.

13. Lerman BB, Belardinelli L, West GA, et al. Adenosine-sensitive ventricular tachycardia: evidence suggesting cyclic AMP-mediated triggered activity. Circulation 1986;74(2):270–80.

14. Hayashi H, Fujiki A, Tani M, et al. Role of sympathovagal balance in the initiation of idiopathic ventricular tachycardia originating from right ventricular outflow tract. Pacing Clin Electrophysiol 1997; 20(10 Pt 1):2371–7.

15. Krittayaphong R, Bhuripanyo K, Punlee K, et al. Effect of atenolol on symptomatic ventricular arrhythmia without structural heart disease: a randomized placebo-controlled study. Am Heart J 2002;144(6):e10.

16. Gill JS, Mehta D, Ward DE, et al. Efficacy of flecainide, sotalol, and verapamil in the treatment of right ventricular tachycardia in patients without overt cardiac abnormality. Br Heart J 1992;68(4): 392–7.

17. Belhassen B, Rotmensch HH, Laniado S. Response of recurrent sustained ventricular tachycardia to verapamil. Br Heart J 1981;46(6):679–82.

18. Ward DE, Nathan AW, Camm AJ. Fascicular tachycardia sensitive to calcium antagonists. Eur Heart J 1984;5(11):896–905.

19. Chimienti M, Cullen MT Jr, Casadei G. Safety of long-term flecainide and propafenone in the management of patients with symptomatic paroxysmal atrial fibrillation: report from the Flecainide and Propafenone Italian Study Investigators. Am J Cardiol 1996;77(3):60A–75A.

20. Morady F, Kadish AH, DiCarlo L, et al. Long-term results of catheter ablation of idiopathic right ventricular tachycardia. Circulation 1990;82(6): 2093–9.

21. Tanawuttiwat T, Nazarian S, Calkins H. The role of catheter ablation in the management of ventricular tachycardia. Eur Heart J 2016;37(7):594–609.

22. Ling Z, Liu Z, Su L, et al. Radiofrequency ablation versus antiarrhythmic medication for treatment of ventricular premature beats from the right ventricular outflow tract: prospective randomized study. Circ Arrhythm Electrophysiol 2014;7(2): 237–43.

23. Latchamsetty R, Yokokawa M, Morady F, et al. Multicenter outcomes for catheter ablation of idiopathic premature ventricular complexes. J Am Coll Cardiol: Clin Electrophysiol 2015;1(3):116–23.

24. Coggins DL, Lee RJ, Sweeney J, et al. Radiofrequency catheter ablation as a cure for

idiopathic tachycardia of both left and right ventricular origin. J Am Coll Cardiol 1994;23(6):1333–41.

25. Nakagawa H, Beckman KJ, McClelland JH, et al. Radiofrequency catheter ablation of idiopathic left ventricular tachycardia guided by a Purkinje potential. Circulation 1993;88(6):2607–17.

26. Lin D, Hsia HH, Gerstenfeld EP, et al. Idiopathic fascicular left ventricular tachycardia: linear ablation lesion strategy for noninducible or nonsustained tachycardia. Heart Rhythm 2005;2(9): 934–9.

27. Wen MS, Yeh SJ, Wang CC, et al. Radiofrequency ablation therapy in idiopathic left ventricular tachycardia with no obvious structural heart disease. Circulation 1994;89(4):1690–6.

28. Yamada T, McElderry HT, Doppalapudi H, et al. Focal ventricular tachycardia arising from the epicardial crux of the heart after a remote inferior myocardial infarction. J Cardiovasc Electrophysiol 2009;20(8):944–5.

29. Sadek MM, Benhayon D, Sureddi R, et al. Idiopathic ventricular arrhythmias originating from the moderator band: electrocardiographic characteristics and treatment by catheter ablation. Heart Rhythm 2015;12(1):67–75.

30. Santoro F, DI Biase L, Hranitzky P, et al. Ventricular tachycardia originating from the septal papillary muscle of the right ventricle: electrocardiographic and electrophysiological characteristics. J Cardiovasc Electrophysiol 2015;26(2):145–50.

31. Doppalapudi H, Yamada T, McElderry HT, et al. Ventricular tachycardia originating from the posterior papillary muscle in the left ventricle: a distinct clinical syndrome. Circ Arrhythm Electrophysiol 2008;1(1):23–9.

32. Tada H, Ito S, Naito S, et al. Idiopathic ventricular arrhythmia arising from the mitral annulus: a distinct subgroup of idiopathic ventricular arrhythmias. J Am Coll Cardiol 2005;45(6):877–86.

33. Tada H, Tadokoro K, Ito S, et al. Idiopathic ventricular arrhythmias originating from the tricuspid annulus: prevalence, electrocardiographic characteristics, and results of radiofrequency catheter ablation. Heart Rhythm 2007; 4(1):7–16.

34. Van Herendael H, Garcia F, Lin D, et al. Idiopathic right ventricular arrhythmias not arising from the outflow tract: prevalence, electrocardiographic characteristics, and outcome of catheter ablation. Heart Rhythm 2011;8(4):511–8.

35. Kawamura M, Gerstenfeld EP, Vedantham V, et al. Idiopathic ventricular arrhythmia originating from the cardiac crux or inferior septum: epicardial idiopathic ventricular arrhythmia. Circ Arrhythm Electrophysiol 2014;7(6):1152–8.

36. Mountantonakis SE, Frankel DS, Tschabrunn CM, et al. Ventricular arrhythmias from the coronary

venous system: prevalence, mapping, and ablation. Heart Rhythm 2015;12(6):1145–53.

37. Doppalapudi H, Yamada T, Ramaswamy K, et al. Idiopathic focal epicardial ventricular tachycardia originating from the crux of the heart. Heart Rhythm 2009;6(1):44–50.

38. Katz DF, Turakhia MP, Sauer WH, et al. Safety of ventricular tachycardia ablation in clinical practice: findings from 9699 hospital discharge records. Circ Arrhythm Electrophysiol 2015;8(2): 362–70.

39. Peichl P, Wichterle D, Pavlu L, et al. Complications of catheter ablation of ventricular tachycardia: a single-center experience. Circ Arrhythm Electrophysiol 2014;7(4):684–90.

40. Tan AY, Hu YL, Potfay J, et al. Impact of ventricular ectopic burden in a premature ventricular contraction-induced cardiomyopathy animal model. Heart Rhythm 2016;13(3):755–61.

41. Latchamsetty R, Bogun F. Premature ventricular complexes and premature ventricular complex induced cardiomyopathy. Curr Probl Cardiol 2015; 40(9):379–422.

42. El Kadri M, Yokokawa M, Labounty T, et al. Effect of ablation of frequent premature ventricular complexes on left ventricular function in patients with nonischemic cardiomyopathy. Heart Rhythm 2015; 12(4):706–13.

43. O'Donnell D, Cox D, Bourke J, et al. Clinical and electrophysiological differences between patients with arrhythmogenic right ventricular dysplasia and right ventricular outflow tract tachycardia. Eur Heart J 2003;24(9):801–10.

44. Vestal M, Wen MS, Yeh SJ, et al. Electrocardiographic predictors of failure and recurrence in patients with idiopathic right ventricular outflow tract tachycardia and ectopy who underwent radiofrequency catheter ablation. J Electrocardiol 2003; 36(4):327–32.

45. Ito S, Tada H, Naito S, et al. Development and validation of an ECG algorithm for identifying the optimal ablation site for idiopathic ventricular outflow tract tachycardia. J Cardiovasc Electrophysiol 2003; 14(12):1280–6.

46. Sekiguchi Y, Aonuma K, Takahashi A, et al. Electrocardiographic and electrophysiologic characteristics of ventricular tachycardia originating within the pulmonary artery. J Am Coll Cardiol 2005;45(6): 887–95.

47. Joshi S, Wilber DJ. Ablation of idiopathic right ventricular outflow tract tachycardia: current perspectives. J Cardiovasc Electrophysiol 2005; 16(Suppl 1):S52–8.

48. Iwai S, Cantillon DJ, Kim RJ, et al. Right and left ventricular outflow tract tachycardias: evidence for a common electrophysiologic mechanism. J Cardiovasc Electrophysiol 2006;17(10):1052–8.

49. Krittayaphong R, Sriratanasathavorn C, Dumavibhat C, et al. Electrocardiographic predictors of long-term outcomes after radiofrequency ablation in patients with right-ventricular outflow tract tachycardia. Europace 2006;8(8):601–6.

50. Bala R, Garcia FC, Hutchinson MD, et al. Electrocardiographic and electrophysiologic features of ventricular arrhythmias originating from the right/left coronary cusp commissure. Heart Rhythm 2010; 7(3):312–22.

Moving?

Make sure your subscription moves with you!

To notify us of your new address, find your **Clinics Account Number** (located on your mailing label above your name), and contact customer service at:

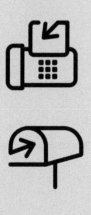

Email: journalscustomerservice-usa@elsevier.com

800-654-2452 (subscribers in the U.S. & Canada)
314-447-8871 (subscribers outside of the U.S. & Canada)

Fax number: 314-447-8029

Elsevier Health Sciences Division
Subscription Customer Service
3251 Riverport Lane
Maryland Heights, MO 63043

*To ensure uninterrupted delivery of your subscription, please notify us at least 4 weeks in advance of move.